THE TWISTED LOVE OF FOOD ADDICTION

Releasing Your Pounds of Pain

Echo Laymon Pelster

Copyright © 2022 by Echo Laymon Pelster.

All Rights Reserved. No part of this publication may be reproduced, distributed, or transmitted in any form or by any means, including photocopying, recording, or other electronic or mechanical methods, or by any information storage and retrieval system without the prior written permission of the publisher, except in the case of very brief quotations embodied in critical reviews and certain other noncommercial uses permitted by copyright law.

ISBN: 979-8-218-06801-1

DEDICATION

For My Aunt Mary – The North Star a Guiding Light For My Life.

For Vern and Cash Dog; The Special Lights in My Life.

For Our Children, Whom Will See Clearly in their own time.

Remembering those who transitioned in tragedy, remembering that no one truly dies.

For all my readers, written from the heart because I don't know any other way to do it.

A free Bonus Gift to you: EchoPelsterSpeaks.com Under Freebies

ECHOPELSTERSPEAKS.COM

Echo Laymon Pelster *www.echopelsterspeaks.com*

ABOUT THE AUTHOR

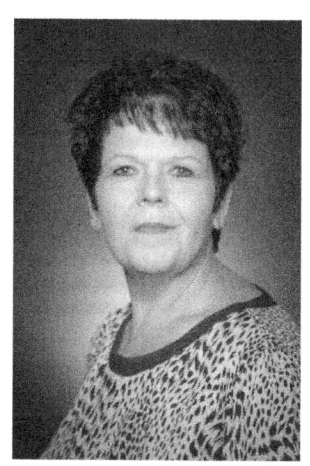

Echo Laymon Pelster is an International Best- Selling Amazon Author, Keynote Speaker, and Certified Methodology Transformational Trainer, Barrett Values Certified Leadership Coach, she successfully helps clients in every culture breakthrough business & personal weight-loss barriers, self-imposed limitations by inspiring self-care, masterful methodology, self-confidence, with consciousness in spiritual health.

Echo knows that obesity has less to do with what people are eating and more to do with what is eating them.

Through education and inspiration, she brings value to individuals, organizations, institutions, patient aftercare corporate and medical organizations in support of their procedures and practices.

She is also aware that how a person does one thing they likely do everything. There are 7 core areas in life, and she knows the value of tying it all together. Grounding the individual in all areas of life.

Aware of how obese people cope, isolate, and hide out, Echo knows that the weight is only a mere distraction, I help them get out of the obesity trap, most obese people likely use food as their source of love and protection, buffering the real issues and creating the burial of the truest desires and emotions, this false appetite leaves the obese person and the binge eater compulsively hungry, sometimes food addicted and personally lost.

It is the same thread that pulls the workaholic, over-enthusiastic exercise enthusiast, or anyone else who is compulsively obsessed and acting out to avoid emotions. From food addictions to gambling the principles she teaches work, privately and without judgment.

Obesity is a health concern behind the desk, further stress slows release. My interest peaked when I discovered colleagues were uninsurable because of height and build issues.

Her professional experience includes over 41 years in direct sales, including financial services with Thrivent, Principal & New York Life. Echo is certified in several areas in Financial Services including RICP, CTLC, FIC, and CDFA, and is currently finishing her ChFC.

Echo is Certified in several breakthrough modalities and coaching methods to get the highest results. With over 41 years in sales with accolades that include Pinnacle Performance 2017, Balanced Practice 2021, and Coaching others to success, and now Echo shares what she has learned, how the learning has brought insight into her life, and how she knows anyone can thrive no matter what has happened to them, what others have done to them, or how they coped and abused themselves.

Echo lives in the heart of the Sandhills of Nebraska with her husband LaVern of 25 years and enjoys writing, live and virtual speaking events, one-on-one coaching, and walking their dog, Cash.

"When I had my first gastric bypass, I believed it would make me thin forever. Afterward, I weighed over 357 pounds, so I had another, lost 203 pounds, and made the local paper…only to gain back more than 114 pounds. Ashamed, isolated, and hiding out, I discovered principles to lose and keep the weight off."

Email:

echopelster@echopelsterspeaks.com | www.echopelsterspeaks.com

Echo is an International Best-Selling Amazon Author and one of America's Most Sought After Keynote Speakers Internationally offering only 40 dates each Year in The Book on Transformation available on www.EchoPelsterSpeaks.com Email Echo at Echo-Pelster@EchoPelsterSpeaks.com

THE TWISTED LOVE OF FOOD ADDICTION

CONTENTS

CHAPTER ONE
We can only learn what we are taught, by circumstances or others. 1

CHAPTER TWO
Throw Away Child: You Throw Away the First Child Just Like You Give the First Pancake to the Dog. 9

CHAPTER 3
My Spirituality Became Broken at Church. 30

CHAPTER 4
Broken Promises: We Stop Believing When No One Follows Through. 43

CHAPTER 5 IDENTITY THEFT
You are confined only by the walls you build yourself - Unknown 58

CHAPTER 6 LITTLE JOE
Trust cannot live in the same space as secrets and lies. 67

CHAPTER 7
The Murder of Bucky 80

CHAPTER 8
Alleged Right of a Parent 88

CHAPTER 9
Shot and Raped 97

CHAPTER 10
    Stepfather's Death in My Playhouse! *101*

CHAPTER 11:
    Given to Strangers *112*

CHAPTER 12
    Forever Different the New Awareness *126*

CHAPTER 13 KEEP THE CHANGE
    How Intervention Saved My Life *159*

CHAPTER 14
    Releasing the Pounds of Pain *173*

CHAPTER 15
    If I feel my Emotions I will fall apart, Barbie is plastic, I am not *178*

CHAPTER 16
    What I Learned & You can too! *191*

EPILOGUE
    The Ego and the Soul *205*

Echo Laymon Pelster *www.echopelsterspeaks.com*

HOW TO USE THIS BOOK

Every Chapter has stories reactions and solutions that the Author used to overcome food addiction, every chapter end has questions to ask yourself, don't hurry through, answer, and write about every question that resonates with you or that you identify with.

Maybe you will treat yourself to a new journal as you celebrate the fact that you are not alone and the feeling that other people feel just like you, you just haven't met these new friends yet.

The author started her recovery story in her early 20s and overcame addictive eating after even two gastric bariatric surgeries did not solve her problem.

There is hope for you too! You are not alone, I am here! Right with you on every page, the good news is today I have a choice, and you can too.

Much love, Echo

CHAPTER ONE

We can only learn what we are taught, by circumstances or others.

The unexpected is the great teacher of flexibility, adaptability, and trust.
- Gary Zukav

Perception is everything, this book is written from my perception, I expect that other family members would see this differently or remember it differently, but that truly does not matter, often two people can be at the same event and have a different experience.

This book is about my emotional journey, how I felt, what happened, the words I heard with my ears, what happened and how I perceived the events that lead to devastation, grief, and obesity.

This book is also about my own recovery from compulsive overeating and has lots of tips, tricks, and thought nuggets that will allow you to overcome eating what you don't want to eat also. I know that people know what to eat. But imagine, what if it's not what you are eating, but what is eating you?

My perception is not debatable or wrong not even less real, it's just my perception, what I saw, heard, and felt, and what happened to my own inner voice of knowing who I was in the process.

How I Packed on over 200 pounds that I didn't need in a desperate lifestyle of compulsive eating and was frozen into an existence where all I really wanted was to feel love, be loved.

How it benefited and kept me safe until it no longer worked and held me back until I could sort out my own truth with my own intuition, spiritually, and DNA.

How I discovered the defining moments that brought me to the realization that I must be the master of my own fate and guide my ship to my life's port, happiness, and purposeful destiny.

It's easy to imagine things as a child when adults are not truthful when you are a smart little kid and can identify a lie quickly you lose trust in those who are supposed to love you and care for you most, I did.

It's easy to be afraid as a child when the rules change each day, and actions that were okay yesterday are a crime today, my childhood was unpredictable, chaotic, and often confusing.

I remember myself as a lonely, unwanted child, unloved child, I didn't have a lot of friends and my one true friend moved away when we were in the first grade, but she is still a dear friend, we got together from time to time in life, and we always remember how happy we were when we were together back in the 1960s.

My Feelings were always the first thing that was undermined at our house, I was not to have feelings, express feelings, or show feelings, and Lord knows I was not allowed to tell anyone about my feelings that was a never rule. So, I never told my feelings to anyone, they were a part of my family's secret-keeping, we pretend everything is wonderful no matter what, we didn't want the neighbors or the world to know the truth, not our teachers or the people at church.

It's easy to justify your choices when they are designed to benefit yourself and not the greater good of all household members.

I felt like a little slave at a young age and I didn't even know it, I worked hard and did a good job cleaning the living room so hopefully, mom would love me, if I didn't she didn't, her approval was my reward for a job well done, I thought every child worked hard to get to eat, have a place to sleep, and be warm, I didn't know other parents provided that, and their kids did chores because it was a part of being a family and cleaning up together, I was just given work to do, never shown how to do anything, and if it wasn't right I got to do it over till it was perfect enough for that day, other day's it may have never been perfect enough. And other days it may not have even been required.

What I learned is what others accused me of is what they were doing themselves, there was always a double standard and a double rule for everything. Even different rules for different kids.

Chaos and confusion were the norms for me. How I perceived the actions of those around me had everything to do with everything. Our perception has everything to do with everyone.

I discovered that the only one who ever needed to keep promises was me. I'm glad I learned that, and today I am keeping my promise to myself by writing to you and the rest of the world, so you can know you are not alone, and all suffering can be overcome.

Did you ever get to the end of your day and wonder, where did the day go, and then realize you had not kept your word in so many areas that it was overwhelming to think about what you were behind on? Me too.

When I made a promise to myself and did not keep it when I said I would do something for someone else, I am agreeing with myself first before I was agreeing with others, first with myself, and then with others.

When I commit to something with someone else, I make the agreement with myself first. I decide I am going to do something, then I speak it aloud with a yes to someone else.

And when I don't keep my promise, my commitments, or my word, I lose face with others, myself, and with my own soul, when I no longer trust myself to follow through with things I no longer participate in life, I become isolated, I had lost my trust in myself and I no longer believed in myself, I become embarrassed, I was ashamed, I hid out and I emotionally disappeared from myself. And I really did not know why, and then I found out.

Just as the phoenix rises out of the ashes and has new birth, so can you and I, the ashes keep our skin young and vibrant, they remind us we are alive, in all pain, discomfort, and simple pleasures, as we rise out of the ashes, we take our life back.

When we do not keep our promises to our children, we lose credibility with our children and it costs us their respect, when we fail to keep our promises to ourselves, we lose our self-confidence in every area of our life. We lose faith in many people, places things, and ideas. We lose our emotional mastery, of knowing ourselves, and the truth, the truth of our birthright, whom we were intended to become and born to be.

I often hear people say, my kids are a handful, and I just can't handle them. Often my response is how often do you keep your word and follow through? When we don't follow through with our children, we lose their trust and respect.

Children believe there is something wrong with them and you don't love them if you don't take your time to be with them, or chose to spend time with them, kids don't need a phone, tv, or game box, they need a tackle box, conversation, family fun, meals where parents sit down with them and take time to talk to them, and only you can make time for them.

Hanging out with your kids will be one of the most important things you will do, if you didn't have that as a child you may be like I was and not know how, now with your own children, looking back however I realize it was not a skill I had to learn just something I needed to do.

It is the same with us, every time we tell ourselves we are going to eat right, and exercise and we don't do it we are breaking down our own self-respect subconsciously, and minimizing our own self-confidence a little bit more each time we do not follow through, or our actions are not in alignment with what we say we want, so we don't believe ourselves or take our dreams and goals seriously, or take the words we say to ourselves seriously, I didn't believe myself any longer.

I was exactly lost in how I looked and believed that my state of obesity was my value and my destiny; at 357.8 pounds I didn't even see myself as fat. I was not seeing myself in the mirror the way I looked, or as others saw me, people would say things like, she really has a beautiful face but…she really ought to do something with her weight.

I put on my oversized clothes and tried to hide myself and my body, as though something that large could be hidden, and make-up was a must, I couldn't be a messy or slobby-looking fat person, but I was deep inside, that's how I felt about myself and I didn't even realize that was the message that I was giving to myself, and I remained hidden behind the mask and garb, never truly seeing my actual size and reality until one day I did.

When I finally faced the number on the scale it was devastating, I had done all the right things, read all the right books, tried all the popular diets, read all the food information, macronutrients, sugar busters, you name it, I had gone to overeaters anonymous only to not identify with eating M&M's off the floor or stealing someone else's lunch, I didn't fit in anywhere, my conditioning was such that I decided to look outside of myself for the answers and I found out the answers were not there either.

I had the first gastric bypass at age 24 when I was only 224 pounds so my weight would not skyrocket out of control, no one ever talked to me about holistic nutrition, realistic expectations, or aftercare for myself other than seeing a gastric specialist once each year, so the bypass didn't solve my weight problem, and here I was 357.8 pounds at 37 years old, with congestive heart failure symptoms and pulmonary hypertension.

Desperately looking for a solution, taking on the guilt of managing my own self-care, deep-down knowing I was not really in alignment with what needed to be done, what did I do?

I did what I thought would be the easiest softest way and realistically thought it was a silver bullet cure to my weight and eating issues, I took the doctor's suggestion to have a second gastric bypass, the first one just wasn't the right type for my body type, that's why it wasn't successful, or so I thought at the time, so I chose to have a new gastric Roux, and Y gastric procedure that would almost kill me.

I truly believed the first time as well as the second time that the gastric bypass would make me thin forever, it would stop me from eating and be the cure of all cures. I really was not telling myself the truth that my eating was how I was coping with what was happening in my past subconscious childhood life, or in the failure to align my thoughts, words, deeds, and actions here and now.

Insanity is doing the same thing repeatedly expecting a different outcome.

With the second gastric bypass, this time I lost 203 pounds in about 2 years, was a local celebrity, inspired others to have the procedure due to the article in our local paper, spent over $20,000 on plastic surgery to remove the skin, felt great, and gained back over 114 pounds only to become lost again.

It wasn't what I was eating it was what was eating me, it was my family's rejection, emotionally devastating hurts, the death of four of my siblings and two failed marriages, unfaithful spouses', personal losses, and the promises to myself that remained undone that were incompletes in my life like the homework a child fails to turn in.

If you are ready to change your life you will find my story helpful, my story will resonate with you whether you are currently thick or thin.

And I will love and accept you through your process of finding out how you will lose your pounds of pain whether they are physical or emotional.

I will help you rethink your beliefs and get in touch with your personal self-value, worthiness, and your emotional higher self and real values.

I will challenge you to think, about the stories you were told and the stories you have told yourself, on your own terms, we are going for the gold.

We are working to find out who you are in this book. Find out who you want to be, and who you can be! Finding out for yourself once and for all, the treasures that you hold within yourself, that make you who you are and who you were truly born to be, and the only permission you will ever need is your own.

Who are you? What were you put on earth for? And where are you going from here? I know you want to know. I did.

And it changed my life and brought me to my natural weight. Where the mind goes the body follows, today I am grateful for all the discomfort, sadness, grief, and unhappiness I came through, it makes me who I am, and I have an awesome life and truly enjoy happiness. With a vibrant life, lots of friends, travel, joy, love, and abundance, I love living today.

QUESTIONS TO ASK YOURSELF & Journal About:

Do I remember the "first time" of realizing that eating felt good,

not because I am hungry, but because I was hurt? Who was involved in the event?

Was it something I told myself, or did someone else tell me? Is it true?

Did I hide it or keep it a secret? Why did I do that? Have you ever eaten in secret?

Why did you hide eating?

Did someone make you feel shame for eating? Who?

Why did it hurt you?

CHAPTER TWO

Throw Away Child: You Throw Away the First Child Just Like You Give the First Pancake to the Dog.

Be mindful of what you throw away, and whom you push away, and be careful of what you walk away from.

-Unknown

I will bet you without a doubt that getting fat and becoming overweight or morbidly obese was not something you daydreamed about doing as a child, I am pretty sure it was not on your bucket list unless you were seeking the world book of Guinness records or possibly you desired to become a Sumo wrestler.

Me either.

But it happened I didn't have a clue how to stop it, I tried to eat right and exercise and always found myself ruining the day with a dear friend Little Debbie, a Snack named Snickers, or a pound of the cheapest cookies I could afford, in those days, always in the mid-afternoon, binging on candy bars and hiding sugary snacks from my family, keeping my additive treats secret and available, but only for me, as though they didn't see them hanging off of my body in the pounds of fat.

As a child I was told I should expect to be obese because most everyone was, other family members believed they were born to be obese, and so I believed through their words and conditioning that I was born to be obese because they all were they were told they would be, and they were, the belief fulfilled their destiny, they called it the Laymon curse, a lie we as a family told ourselves to justify our bad eating habits, like eating a whole pie as a snack yet some family members declared we had an undiagnosed thyroid problem, or hidden from science glandular disorder, nope, how about a distorted health value system and values that were not in alignment with the things we professed we wanted.

The truth hurts, but not every single person in the family was fat, none of them were truly obese children looking back at the family pictures all of them were prescribed the obesity formula because the parents or grandparents became obese, but it was not caused by anything genetic, it was caused faulty belief systems, unreasonable folklore, and by sugar, foods that come in wrappers and rich dairy laden fatty foods and sauces.

In my late teens, I had already learned how to tell the story of how I would be fat like my parents and paternal grandparents, it was generational, and I did not believe I had a choice about my own body, I was preconditioned by the idea from my mother, she expected me to be a fat slob like my dad, and later by the words of my father's family anytime the subject came up.

I believed people would just believe me and they would think I was just naturally overweight, it wasn't how I saw myself or how I wanted to be, and it wasn't how I wanted to be seen. It was how it was. I truly believed I had no choice in the matter whatsoever.

The biggest lies I told were the ones I told myself because I was the only one who believed them anyway. I did not even investigate the things my family said to me, I just gullibly believed what I was told through my childhood and young adult years, I believed that if a family member told me something they told me to help me, however when I went out into the world, I found myself more than once embarrassed, and questioned by others about where my thinking came from and why.

The events of the past and the truth of our perception of that past, almost always step on the heels of the future until the old stories are rewritten and resolved until they can no longer creep in and take over the intentions of the person who is trying to become aware of the real truth and overcome old teachings that suited and served the people telling the original stories, but these subconscious things are not so obvious, and to change them, when they are remembered, to bring them to resolution and re-write them as they are dissolved from constant memory and powerlessness so they can now fade away, they will be a memory but only a memory of usefulness in your life's learning process, not a memory that creates hurt, pain, anxiety, poor self-esteem, unconscious self-sabotage, numbness, and hopelessness.

Changing these old records and rewriting our future is a powerful, and conscious decision that we always have a choice about. Consciously changing the actions, we take and overcoming the things that hold us back, breaking away from our previous patterns, and the expectations of others, and having realistic expectations for ourselves are the freedom that will bring us to our own happiness and lasting change.

Daydreaming and looking for memories of hope was what I first became grateful for, that brought me enormous strength, unconditional kindness, reciprocal meaningful love, exuberant joy, and incredible self-worthiness, that has allowed me to become more than what I was ever told I could be, more than I ever dared to imagine, that's what happened to me when I cleared my mind and opened my heart.

I found my family and support system, not the people I was born to, but the family in the world, I could identify with and resonate with in times of challenge because my biological family was emotionally absent, controlling, and often left me feeling like I was nothing.

As a child I did not fit in, as an adult, I didn't measure up because I grew up and started to question the holy grail belief systems I was raised under and that was like blasphemy against the family code and God somehow.

As a young adult, I would cry all the way home hoping it would be different this trip, and then cry all the way back to my home again with anger at myself for being such a fool, hoping something changed and their hearts and love for me, compassion, and kindness for me, I had unreal expectations they taught me that I could not make them, my family more than they chose to be. But I could choose.

The truth was my people could not give me what they did not possess. Eventually, I stopped making the trip after the death of my grandparents because it was just too painful, and hurtful to be disrespected in such an overwhelming way, and I couldn't stand the dysfunction and the lies.

When someone shows you who they are, believe them, and don't go back for repeated hurt and pain, if there is anything there for you, they will reach out with positive action and then you can decide. My immediate family never reached out, the road only ran from my direction to their world to them, never from their world to mine, the phone never rang, and any calls made were from me to them, in other word's they never did show up in my life.

I will hang my hat and go to the places, where I am celebrated, not just tolerated. My value is not determined by their neglect. Criticism or Opinion. But I didn't know that I had to learn that.

Memories are tricky and sticky things, that have their own twists and turns, some memories are true, others are lies we have either told ourselves or been told by others, I had to investigate within the stillness of myself, through the validation of others and investigate the stories of what I was told.

I found my own answers, and in the process, I had to admit what parts were troubles I created for myself, what was someone else's that was not mine to wear, claim, or clean up, and what was important and mattered and what didn't matter at all.

What luggage of the past was I still carrying around unnecessarily, in the form of weight on my mind, that resulted in the obesity in my body?

What I had continued to drag around like a sack of rocks, the pounds, and pounds of painful memories that no longer served a purpose, they were and are important clearing and tasking, painfully and shockingly, moving them out of the darkness into truth and light.

I had to let go of those pet rocks which had their own names of shame, blame, and anger, I had to take responsibility for my part in every part of my life and allow true awareness to be revealed in thought processes to live openly, be honest with no regrets, and allow myself to be celebrated as a part of the natural path to personal human experience and wholeness.

Seeking out where something started can be valuable and insightful. But it can also be scary and daunting, often becoming the things we hide, whether ourselves or through other people's secrets.

What was said to me and how I heard it can be quite another. Re- examining conversational memory can be gracious or vicious, depending on how you remember or heard the sentence.

Perception in our life events is exactly that, if we are upset about another person's words or behavior as an adult and tell no one our feelings then we are at fault. We are expected to be proactive, however, when an adult was frozen as a child, not allowed to speak or have opinion, the adult doesn't know how to respond.

If we are a child and are scolded for asking, wanting, or needing and we learn it is not safe to ask, that is quite another, the character defect is with the adult, not the child.

I was the oldest of 8 children with the first 5 being born in less than 6 years. Of the first five, children, we had four different fathers. Between the eight of us children, we had 6 different fathers.

My mother did not like to talk to me or answer my questions, I was to be out of sight and out of mind where she was concerned, she didn't want me there, and I was forced out of her sight in most situations which included being locked in my room, locked out of the house in severely hot weather with no water source, or grounded for months at a time, I learned to enjoy her punishment of isolation where I could live how I wanted, at least in my imagination, and because she considered me a trouble maker she allowed my younger sisters to play in the house under a cool fan, me with no toys to play with, often I was left with huge grocery boxes of green beans to stem, where I sat in the shade and worked, I imagined myself as Cinderella, and Rogers and Hammerstein were going to find me someday and make me beautiful, skinny and famous. I was lonely and put into slavery quite young.

I was always hushed, told to find something to do and leave my mother alone. I felt unwanted because my mother was not shy about telling me I was unwanted, she considered me as though I was the first pancake in the batch, the one you throw away.

I am sure they would tell you I was wanted but it never felt that way, as an empath I could feel everything other people around me felt, every person's expressions, the emotional state they were in and their words, I knew who was saying what to me by the emotions that were pouring out of them, the words I heard and what I felt was totally different, today I realize this is an inborn gift that I could not recognize and appreciate until I was older, once I became aware of it, I learned to appreciate it and respect it equally.

Emotional energy does not lie, we are connected to it and by it, and we can feel it if we are looking for it in every conversation, I can also tell a bullshitter right off. This makes the hairs on the back of my neck stand up. I have learned to listen to my God Given Antennas and I hope that you will too.

By the time I was in my thirties four of my siblings were dead, none of them of natural causes, all of them died of horrific tragic events that would change my life and how I saw the adults in my life forever.

I was so emotionally in touch with how others felt, I could feel their pain, when they died and how they died. My Emotions and memories are frozen in the horror of their tragic end in my own reality. It was as though I could feel it. I had learned to expect the worst because it kept happening.

I often knew they were dead before my phone rang for someone to tell me. It was as strange for me to experience as for you reading about it, I am sure, I kept the secret for many years, worrying what others would think if they knew, I knew, or if they realized

I could feel with an uncanny since even the simplest omissions, deceptions, and the tiniest of lies.

I know I had young parents who escaped from whatever life they started in, I am glad they escaped, whether real or imagined, unfortunately, I was their hostage.

In my mother's case, she hated her mother so anything that her mother suggested in my interest she would do exactly the opposite of what was suggested by my grandmother, and my father I think was just young and dumb and caught in the middle as I was.

Unfortunately for my father, he was my mother's escape route to get away from home, my mother got pregnant, and I guess she was thinking free, I never really saw it that way, my mother had someone's baby every year for years, hardly freedom.

Watching my mother's life in my childhood made me not really want to ever have a family, I did of course, but it wasn't a focused want. It was a traditional generational accident that's been going on in families for generations. Having children should always be a choice. Not an expectation.

Looking back and seeing all the defects of the character that my father may have portrayed in his youth and early adult years, he was still the most decent man my mother ever married, but when you put two people who are just like one another in a cage together it gets pretty gnarly, and it was, they were both violent and hateful toward each other, but I am sure it didn't start that way, after all, I am here, and I have a sister fathered by the same man, my dad, and rumor has it back in the day they acted like a couple of rabbits.

I am lucky I didn't have big ears.

History has proven that so many of the most brutal crimes were born out of lust, then betrayal, then hate because of the emotional hurt and pain, and many of those old stories ended in murder.

There is nothing new under the sun, just new stories with different faces and places in them. That's my parents, just a different face and a different place, as I have aged, I can see that.

But when it was all happening, it felt like the whole world could see us, as though we lived and a glass house, and it felt like they knew everything too.

As a result, my parents should have been required to take lessons before having children, for my sake, I was and am a soft-hearted person and I suffered greatly at their hands, or at the lack of their hands, I was neglected and alone in a large family, I really don't think they got out of bed each morning with the intentions of doing me emotional harm on any day in the life, I think they were so wrapped up in their own drama they could not see me wilting away, internalizing, feeling lost, losing trust, and cautious of even of their behavior, towards me, the neighbors or even themselves, I was a child that sensed the motives in what they did and what they failed to do, as a child, I didn't trust adults, they had let me down, they lied, they didn't keep their promises, and they always said if I was good they would do something special and it never happened, if I cleaned my room something good would happen and it never did.

Adults became liars in our house, I was angry that they lied, and I was always sent to my room especially when I pointed out their lies which left me always alone. I lived in a do as I say world, not as I do.

I didn't even know I remembered some of the horrible things that happened in my life, partially because of the fact that our normal was not like other people's normal, but my body and subconscious mind remembered, I would often set my goal to start a new diet and lose weight only to plummet by the end of the morning, afternoon, or end of the day, I didn't have a clue why, when I started looking for the truth, I realized I had to find out who I was and find myself first and foremost, what I truly wanted when I started looking out of the box and seeking answers that would help me realign my life, the words who am I, and what do I want were some of the hardest words I ever asked myself.

Who are you? What do you want?

I started to learn about my subconscious mind which decides nearly every trajectory of life prior to age nine, which is influenced by absolutely everything it hears, sees, and receives, every action and every reaction which really does create beliefs, habits, and thinking patterns as a result of that early childhood input most of which had to be and seemed like most had to be reprogramed and re-programming my mind and what it receives for messages within my inner Guidance System.

Learning and knowing it is one thing, recognizing it is another, and changing it is still another.

I have no memories of my mother doing anything with me that was unique or special to me, my liking or enjoyment, my existence or my idea, she taught my other sisters to sew, or garden, or something, but I was the one that she said was too stupid to bother with and she meant it, and I believed it and that was how it was.

More than anything in the world I wanted my mother to love me, talk to me, and just be with me, her pushing me away was a constant in my life, and later in life when I asked her why she said it was my fault, my personality, she just didn't like me, and she never wanted to see me ever again. So far, she hasn't, she will be 80 this year.

I secretly hoped and prayed she could accept me to be her daughter, forgiveness, and happiness would happen between us and change the end of this story. Not so much, I can only want for others what I want for myself, but in some ways, I must always admit where I am powerless. I continue to learn when other people show me who they are, I believe them.

Obviously, I am not stupid, never was, but I had to debunk that message at some point and realize how naïve I was to accept the words of others so willingly, Mother never read books or did coloring, never went to the park, we did go to the fair, and the race horses but I have no special I love you memories from my mom other than one time a song I liked was on the radio and she called me into the kitchen to listen to it, but then I had to go right back to my room where I spent a good portion of my childhood in solitary confinement.

My father was absent for the most part and when he did show up in those days, he was scary, he was mostly scary because my mother told me horror stories about him, so my expectations of him were scary.

Mom taught me fear, fear became like a thief with endless patience in my life, casually circling me like a big ugly bird around my head, it knew I could not guard against it, and eventually, it would catch me off guard when I let my door unlatched, it was what she would do to me, and it taught me to be afraid of my dad, when dad came around my dad and my mother fought a lot, she had boyfriends and he didn't like it, he beat her up, and she beat him back, I watched.

Later she bragged about the wounds she gave him to her friends and us kids and played the victim everywhere else.

I remember her always starting the fight with the words she said, not excusing his behavior, but a lot of it could have been avoided if my mom would have simply shut up or used nicer words and kindness. Mom loved throwing gas on the fire.

My mother wanted to fight, that was her goal. I think that is the part of her that made me a tenacious survivor.

However, I look like my mother and my dad I imagine transfers some of his attitude about her toward me, I feel that often, and if I feel it is probably so.

I know my father does not accept questions well, and his memory is the only memory that is allowed to be validated. I learned not to reminisce about the past with either of my parents. It is out of the safety zone.

We all remember things differently, sometimes because we like to remember things in our favor, sometimes because we really don't remember correctly. But mostly because the memory is distorted or remembered in an attitude or tone that wasn't pleasing to us, or it was pleasing to us, like I said, my memories are my memories, they are attached to how I feel and who I am because of them.

My memories don't define who I am today, however, the truth is sometimes painful instead of happy and sometimes the truth felt too real.

When my father wasn't drinking, I remember he was fun, but I was anxious around him, afraid to be around him alone, I am not exactly sure why, it was an instinct I have, I still have it, and I trust it. Or was it a story was told, I am not sure, either way, I have no real evidence of the feeling's why, so I trust my gut and live in a way that allows me to be present in the moment and safe.

Maybe it was because as a small child I already knew of his unpredictable behavior and worried that someday it would be me getting hit, I was hypervigilant, partially because my mother told me bad things about my dad, which made me afraid of him, and the fights I personally witnessed as a child, however quite honestly.

I have no memories of physical abuse from my dad, but I felt his blows with his words more than once and saw the predicted potential he spoke on my mother through the bruises he left on her, and I saw bruises on other people that declared him the villain.

My instinct was intact I was afraid of him and did not trust him, I didn't know him, and he didn't know me, we are just acquaintances, with no real relational dialog just strangers who have a conversation occasionally, with expected manners from time to time, over my lifetime he is still living, my mother and father are nine days apart in age.

My father didn't act mean and do disgraceful things, when sober but when he drank, he did, I thought of him as a bump, my word as a child for the bum.

My disrespect for my father was taught to me by my mother and corrected with better manners by my grandmother when I told her at a young age my dad was a bump.

I was taught to disrespect the adults my mom didn't like or agree with, and I was expected to respect whoever she did like, and the list changed often, I was confused because I did like some of the people, they treated me nice and noticed me in happy ways, but that was mom's process and it was unpredictable, I gave up people I liked to please my mom, according to her whim on whichever day, gone today, back tomorrow, gone again, often.

I think today that bump was the right word, where my father was concerned, the word is, and was really accurate, and he finally realized years after my parents divorced that his drinking caused bumps in his life and family relationships.

It didn't really change his relationship with me when he quit drinking because he wasn't around, I was kept out of the messiness and no one really talked about, it, unless he got so out of hand, then outsiders or the law, was involved, then it got around more as a rumor. But it was embarrassing and confusing to hear things about your parents that way.

He had unrealistic expectations of instant forgiveness, where many of us were concerned, I gave him acceptance, but I didn't trust him, and I didn't know why, maybe it was because everything that ever happened was somehow everyone else's fault.

Denial of his own past was something my dad did well, he wanted trust he hadn't earned yet.

I didn't know how to talk to him, and he still doesn't know what to say to me, I have tried to have a conversation with him, but doing so was always frustrating and cloudy, he likes to blame, and it's so far gone blame is not an issue, those two people did what they did, they've been divorced well over 50 years and they still use a lot of energy being pissed off at each other, worse yet the other don't even know it, so they could put that energy to more positive use and benefit everyone.

Even as an adult I didn't trust him, today I still have a guarded trust, my dog doesn't like him, and he doesn't have a mean bone in his body, I trust my dog's instincts. I don't know why it is, it just is, it is not something I can fix.

I know my dad made other people's lives hell and again I am glad I didn't have to live in a place where I could feel his rage for my mother, I feel how others feel when they are close by, so I know that stress from the experience.

The stories I often received secondhand of his actions and behavior were unconscionable and unforgivable and since his wife couldn't protect her own children from him, I know with all my heart that his absence from my life was in my best interest. Some wonderful source in the universe saw something bigger and better for me and saved me and I am so grateful.

The children who did live in my dad's house lived what looked like to me a double hell, those kids lived with the biblical rules and people who had the spare, the rod spoil the child justification for the abuse they received, and frankly, that is one of the most ludicrous excuses I have ever heard for the justification of any kind of domestic, gender, racial, hate crimes, or child abuse.

I believe that an eye for an eye creates more blindness, more despair, and more pain, two wrongs have never made anything right that I know of.

I get sick to my stomach when something loving, kind, and joyful is suddenly an excuse that glorifies and justifies the wrongdoing toward others and physically hurting of another life of any kind, human or animal out of sheer cruelty.

I forgive his humanity and how he coped with the woman I called mother, but I do not agree that anyone, anytime had it coming, no matter what their bad acts toward each other were.

What my father did to other people is between him and the people he hurt I don't consider it my business; I don't consider your opinion of me any of my business today either. But I also know that most of the time where there is smoke there is fire, so I tread consciously. Because the Cash Dog knows!

Knowing what he did was shameful and unacceptable and knowing his wife covered it up admittedly left me not trusting her either, my stomach was sickened when she justified his abuse of her children done to them by my father in a conversation, I am glad I had the courageous discussion, she showed me what true co-dependency is, I knew I didn't want any. She inspired me to get a backbone or live in my first crappy marriage, I got my high school diploma, a job and got the heck out of there. Of course, I was in the doghouse for not being a lifer, you know till death do you part. The people that threw that at me the most were divorced justifiably of course. I wasn't in their eyes. They had weak eyes.

Grace kept me out of that situation, and I am grateful even though the only safe place I felt I had been during my childhood was with Grandma and Grandpa. I know they did all they could, but they wanted their own life, they had raised their children and were actively involved a lot, but we were not their kids or responsibility, I often heard the concern in their voices and guidance when they saw us going in a poor direction under parent's neglect and values.

Often it seemed, I was shuffled off to grandma's house so I wouldn't be a nuisance to my mother, this wasn't the first time the universe intervened on my behalf, and I did not know it then, I was too young, but today I am extremely grateful.

I thought grandma and grandpa's house was like my own magic kingdom. There were adventures there, riding to the creek on horseback, shoulder rides, tickling, giggling, and hugs, lots of hugs, and the secret room that contained amazing things for children from Osco drug.

In my Grandparent's house, I was celebrated and loved, corrected as needed, and redirected with learning, conversation, and respect. If I couldn't behave, I had to go lay on the bed and take a nap, I loved that, grandma read books to me after I was there a while, and I really did nap. Her correction was always an experience of learning and love.

I didn't get hugs from my mom, even if she was mean to me all day, I had to give her a kiss on the cheek at night before bed, for me it was a cautious kiss because she was always so angry feeling, there was never any reciprocation whatsoever. She never physically touched me or hugged me, unless she hit me, and that was not a physical touch by her but a stick, belt, or spoon. I craved her love but not her touch. She always bragged that it was legal to use corporal punishment on her kid, ME!

At grandma and grandpa's house in Dumas, I was celebrated, not just tolerated I was totally and always celebrated, we played and drank coffee with grandpa with milk and shudder, my word for sugar.

Dumas Missouri was population 4 back then, Grandma, Grandpa, Aunt Mary, and Uncle Rex, and being with them was like going to heaven, someone bathed me, fed me regular meals, there were treats, car rides, and being pushed on a swing, shoulder rides, eating on the picnic table, feeding birds in homemade milk carton birdhouses, drawing pictures on cardboard and regular naps!

Life for me was amazing at Dumas, when I had a skinned knee there was always a band-aid and a cookie, the cookie was to make my knee feel better, I simply did not know that I was supposed to put my cookie on my knee to make it feel better!

Dumas offered abundant Smouches, kisses, and hugs to make my little life feel better. And then I was returned to my mother, where I was neither seen nor heard, I was invisible, unloved, and lonely.

My mother referred to me as the first pancake in the batch, the one you throw away, or feed the dog. The one that didn't brown right and had no value. I hated that every time she said it. She fed that one to the dog, I was dog food.

If I was sick in the night, I cleaned it up myself, if I was scared, hurt, tired, or had a question I had to figure it out myself, if I needed something, tuff luck kid, money didn't grow on trees, and since your dead-beat dad don't contribute, there might not be enough for the rest of us. My value was based on his payment that she really didn't want, even if he would have paid his child support, I learned that I had no value to either of them.

Later, she acted like dad not paying child support was her decision, "If I take his money, I must take his shit". Nonetheless, I would wake up in the night, puking sick, and go to my mother's room, and either she wasn't there, or she would say get back in bed now, and if I was sick, I had to figure out how to clean the bed, and be well, after all, if I was sick, it was my fault, somehow it was my always my fault.

Neglect taught me to be self-reliant, expect nothing, and ask for nothing. But it also offered me resilience, tenacity and creativity that I might never of had had I been raised with the Cleaver's, Brady's, or Swiss Family Robinson's.

My mother's figure it out for yourself attitude, did make me creative, one time I took the curtains off the window and put them over the vomit spot on my mattress and went back to bed! And I lived!

The attitude of do without simple resources, and neglect also isolated me and made me unsure of myself, sometimes when I had the courage to speak up I was laughed at or made fun of.

Often the opinions of others told me I was doing something wrong even though the truth is that no adult had ever taken the time to teach me how to do it right or at least showed me how they wanted it, but I was expected to know. I was to read minds, be perfect and be telepathic, I think they might have been expecting too much of me. And by the time I was ten I had no expectations anymore. I wanted to run away to Dumas and be a HIPPIE!

One time when I was six years old I broke a glass washing dishes, I was so tired I had been made to re-wash the dishes three or four times that night when I broke the drinking glass I received a bad cut on my left wrist, I still have the scar today, I was paddled with a belt for breaking the glass, my wrist wasn't even a concern till days later when it appeared infected and my mom put bacon grease on it and wrapped it in a torn rag, the whole time telling me that it was my own damned fault, I wasn't more careful, what I knew for sure was the glass was more important than I was, I got the message loud and clear.

In first grade the kids made fun of me with the old rag bandage, I took it off and hid my arm till it was well after that, I took care of myself, washed the grease off with soap and it was better. I don't remember my mom even ever asking me about it again. By now she had 4 little kids younger than me, and I needed to take care of myself.

I was left alone to figure it out. I didn't know how, no one reassured me or told me I could learn how, and I was often told to keep the peace by one adult while another ranted and raved, I was left confused, and scared, and I didn't have the simplest essence of self- confidence I was a little child who felt ugly when she looked in the mirror because her mom said she looked like her dad and she hated him.

Going to Dumas was always amazing to me, Aunt Mary ironed her hair and rolled it on big juice cans, it was fun and magical how she always started out pretty and ended up even prettier, I wanted to be pretty like that, I was 3 or 4 years old, and I didn't believe I was pretty or special at home but at Dumas, I was dressed in nicer clothes and dresses and that felt good.

Aunt Mary was so beautiful and so happy to see me, she has always made a difference in my life with her simple unjudgmental presence. She still does and still is the perfect Aunt, I remember how happy I felt when I was there, with them, it was a magical world for me. I felt so safe there, I didn't really know it or recognize it then, but it was about being so safe, so warm and so loved. It was the one constant I found at Dumas and the people there. It was an amazing revelation when I truly realized it because I could identify a feeling that made sense later on. Even when I pouted and tried to get my own way I was loved and accepted there.

IMPORTANT QUESTIONS TO ASK YOURSELF & Journal About:

How did I seek attention? What did I hide?

How did I hide it?

Why did I hide it?

What are you afraid of?

Who taught you to be afraid?

Did anyone ever tell you to fear another person? Why?

Did it make you afraid of all people who had similar characteristics? Did it make you afraid of Men or Women?

Were you rewarded with food for agreeing with someone? What kind of food was it?

Do you think you are addicted to certain foods? What are they?

What fear comes over you when you think of giving them up?

Are you afraid to cry?

Who taught you to be afraid of your emotions?

Are you ready to feel life yet? Now?

CHAPTER 3

My Spirituality Became Broken at Church.

Religion was invented when the first con man met the first fool
- Mark Twain

At home as a child, I was sent to church with strangers, the church was the free babysitter, and I realize now how naïve I truly was, everyone said going to church was really good for me, but really it was really confusing for me, but it left me well conditioned afraid and unhappy, the stuff they talked about their scared the hell out of me so I am pretty sure that is not where I am going, they made me believe life was to be somber, misery, un-joyful, don't smile, don't be humorous, and be unhappy if I wanted to get to the next life. And by Golly be grateful for it all!

I thought no thanks a lot! I was a child who naturally wanted a more scientific answer, not because I had no faith, but because I needed to connect the dots, I needed it all to make sense, I wanted to understand.

Jesus is another story. His story is the love story of all lives. But only if……….and I already knew I couldn't be good enough to make the cut because I was nobody important enough for someone that good.

Churches filled my head with whom they thought I should become, how I should act or think according to them, and what I should believe. Churches kept me looking for the part of myself that I could not find. That part of me was not there, it was here inside me, just as it is a part of you. The Spirit that lives within You, that is the life force and protection of your own breath, some of us was raised to call it the "holy spirit" in Christianity, but there are many names of it. Definitely Google that.

I remember questioning something at church once, like, their picture of Adam and Eve is white, how did we get black people, and I was told not to question adults!

I think it was among my first abuse and awareness about how I was just to believe what I am told and not think for myself. I remember wanting to debate the issue, I had questions! I needed to understand why it was true, why it wasn't true to me, and if it did why did all this bad stuff happen?

Not one adult sat me down and offered to help me understand, they just pushed their thoughts into my head and down my throat. I became questioning and angry because it did not make sense to me.

My true awareness of how other people fill your head with things that they value and want you to know without your permission, brainwashing comes to mind, some of it became useful and valuable with age and understanding some of it is still nightmare material, some stuff may or may not be of value to me ever.

That answer has left me questioning everything that didn't make sense to me over the rest of my life, if the answer conflicted with the teaching, I was the first kid in the corner every time. I was precocious and curious. I needed you to prove it, I don't remember faith ever being mentioned. If it was, I missed that week.

I questioned how their God only loved some people, and only if they were good enough, I questioned how it could be God made everything and everybody, but he didn't like everyone he made. Seemed odd to me then and doubtful now. It didn't make sense to me, it still doesn't, everyone is in God and God is in everyone. That's my story and I am sticking with it.

I questioned how they knew who wrote their Bible when I learned that most people in that time period couldn't read or write, I questioned why if supposedly God loved everyone, why did they have to do certain rituals for God to love them back, and I really got in the hot soup when I said that I thought God was first, before the bible, the chicken, or the egg!

I wasn't very good at the religious thing as a child, I liked the awards and recognition, and I didn't miss a Sunday for seven years! I still have my Sunday school pins, But I questioned most of what I was being told in one way or another, I felt constantly judged by most of the nice religious people who made sure I knew it.

But mostly I knew I would never be good enough, because of whispers like, don't even have a penny for the plate, dumb as a box of rocks, never enough, poor white trash, and her mother's having another baby, just what they need. I believe that God is Love, and that sure didn't feel loving. I am more valuable than their attitudes and opinions.

Today I realize it probably was not said to me that way or in a tone I imagined, but they were supposed to be nice people and they weren't always nice.

I listened and I don't know that I didn't always know exactly what they were saying really, but I knew and remembered later, particularly the tone in which these self-righteous church people said it. There were nice people and not-so-nice people just like everywhere in the world.

Attention from anyone was important for me because outside of Dumas I didn't get any attention, my food was grains, rice, macaroni, or beans, which I loathe to this day, I was a pudgy little kid but looking back at pictures I have found not fat, not slobby as my mother called me, very normal for my age, most of the communication I received was rather negative and mean, you'd better shut up and eat or else kind of messages. I didn't fall for their God much, but the juice and cookies were good.

Most often I wanted to participate in the fun stuff, so I went along, I got to go to church camp, and I learned to play strip poker there, looking back I laugh, but those counselor people were irate about it. It wasn't something I knew about before I got there. So I can honestly say I went to church to learn poker, strip poker.

I had never played before and never since, but they were pretty pissy about it quite honestly, there we 5 or 6 of us, but for some reason, I was getting the heat, I didn't even own a deck of cards, and besides it made my mother proud, to make my mother proud I always had to do something off-color and out of character, I always ended up feeling ashamed, I think she was the only parent that didn't grab her kid by the ear. But nonetheless, this story is messed up. I am not.

The truth is the truth. I look back and realize there is lots of wisdom to be read including and not limited to only Holy books, personally, I have read it all as an adult with understanding, I often question the translations of how it is interpreted, for me God is bigger than something as petty as a naked butt, or a particular lifestyle it existed before anyone wrote books about it.

And that thing people call God has been around since way before those books were written where a man tried to explain the great power, I choose to call God today, I don't know anyone qualified to write whom God is, as the written word is only as big as the man's mind who wrote it. The Divine One in my mind is limitless.

I had to have a Divine One that was bigger than My life, My thoughts, My Hurts, My Neglect, My Pain, My Parents, Etc. But the whole thing as a kid was something I apparently needed to experience.

I can express how I feel about this great thing, this great power, but I can only tell you about my personal experience with God at my side. I think that's what the people over history were really doing. They wrote down their experiences to give us wonderful spiritual references so we could identify and not feel alone. From this philosophy I am grateful. I can see clearly now.

I was baptized and confirmed, but to this day I am not sure why other than it was something someone else wanted me to do, or I was expected to do, we didn't live it at home, I wanted to be approved of, and if there really was a reason to belong to something I imagine that was what I was seeking, approval, but I remember thinking it was good to be forgiven by someone even though it was someone that I was supposed to see and know in my heart, but even those hugs were often empty and so it all seemed like another phony, thing to cover up how things were.

No amount of church was going to fix what was wrong at our house. At least if the kids were the only ones attending and deciphering the information for themselves, our imaginations were alive and well!

The people at church seemed so perfect to me when I was a child, but we weren't perfect like that at my house. So, I guess in a lot of ways I didn't feel like I fit in there, sometimes I wanted to, but it was more about fitting in and belonging someplace, not worrying about where I might end up later, I never understood going through this life worrying about the next life concepts at all.

I respect other people's choices to do or not do a thing, but I always walked away feeling less than, and not enough, So, each week for years and years I went to church and acted as if everything was okay, but it wasn't.

Then I tried taking what I could swallow and leaving the rest, you might say eating the fish and spitting out the bones, but now I know what's true for me and I do not worry about my next life, I am in a body, it's my meat suit, and when I am done with it, I will go somewhere else, I have a hard time imagining a loving entity that would say they love you with unconditional love and then send you to hell for any reason.

I do not believe that is "God's" way, I do believe that is man's control of another through fear-based leveraging. All great religions of the world have a common denominator, that is to love one another, really that statement right there could bring world peace, religion has started more wars and killed more people than any other cause, so love one another makes sense.

If it's for you, good for you. If it's not there should be no judgment, God existed first, and there are lots of ancient writings like the bible and other holy books.

You have the answers inside you, close your eyes and look around in there, I promise it is all good, all redeemable.

Every person on earth has the right to believe whatever they want. They have the right to believe what is true, what is a lie, and if they like it. Want it, and receive or reject the information in it, then it's yours, your truth, and anything done in love, kindness, and joy, is totally acceptable.

Conditioned Spirits and Learning and conditioning offered to me, by others and their personal beliefs systems, whether generational or traditional, is in no way personal identification, an individual's highest value, or authentic identity of that individual, it has nothing to do with true personal desire or calling, for me it was simply where I was accepted within that particular evolutionary period of time in my own life, I have learned it is neither right nor wrong to choose to leave behind any belief that no longer serves me.

If you are sitting there reading this, and need permission to do the same, Permission Granted, Beliefs separate people, Values bring them closer, and acceptance of one another's differences is the most binding ingredient.

I am who I am, and the approval of others is not a part of the equation today. I seek no approval and try to always do the next right thing.

I don't think in my mind and heart that Jesus ever suggested or intended to be used as a weapon against children by adults to control, suppress or limit their life, he said to love one another. He said to live abundantly. Jesus was just about love, and he went to extremes to prove it!

He did it for the ones who believed themselves unlovable. The poor in spirit. Those who thought something was wrong with them. They are perfect in his eyes and have all the right to live in love, joy, and abundance.

Since there were only synagogues in his time and temples, very few people could read or write, or have resources to write with and on, most of the apostles could not read or write, notedly Peter, the guy put in charge.

It would be fair to assume that the stories changed between storytellers, but in the story of the true love of Jesus Christ, the kind loving man, God's child, just as you are his child, I can bite into that with total belief, the rest of it not so much.

I do believe that how it started and how it was told from generation to generation is like the game we played as children. One person started with a phrase and by the time it got down the row of 20 people the story was different, and whoever wanted the influence knew what to communicate or add to the story to get it.

Control, suppression, and limitations have nothing to do with what God is about. Every person was put on this earth for a purpose, and every life lives and serves accordingly, especially when an individual has the courage to seek through their personal source of power.

Moses did not ever see "GOD" he had a vision of God through the burning bush while on the mountain where he was called to meditate, the bush said I AM is my name, you are the I AM that God was referring to, connected and complete through infinite power who gives you life.

Infinite power is kind, generous, loving, joyful, and helpful and if any person is living a life of love, kindness, and service in abundance and gracious fulfillment, and joy within themselves and bringing that to others, I believe they are in alignment with the great I AM that gives all life breath., you are mirroring the image of God, you are his highest creation, theology, and science support that, we don't need to complicate it by overthinking it, It simply isn't for us to say.

The God I know and understand is not gendered or biased, racially prejudiced, or unhappy with any person or other creation it brought forth.

And you are that creation, God puts no focus on unwanted issues and politics that is man's doing and agenda, nor does God have to explain, God needs no one to explain to the world or the people God created every part of them, every personality, every value, every desire and knowing this everything is perfect.

I am perfect, and so are you, my dreams and aspirations are not only possible, but God allowed the limitless infinite possibilities and if I can hold it in my mind which God inspired then I can accomplish it anywhere and everywhere else, God will reveal the how, and my intuition will reconcile with resolution planning and worthiness because nothing is unworthy. Aspirations are held in the mind of those who live in love and peace. They are for everybody, not just me. Faith that there is something greater than us is all that is needed, we each will latch on to what we need and what we believe is right. But only this great power could do what I could not do for myself.

There is nothing wrong with anything that God made in any way shape or form, all people, places, and things are perfect just as God energy and creation made them, in love, grace, kindness, and joy.

It is not our job, and certainly none of our business to change what was created great! Everything has a purpose, even if it is to show you how you don't want to be, what you don't want to do, or how your actions affect others.

Maybe it is just what you were raised in as your culture, like me, and we followed along like a sheep or cow, you just followed the lead animal because you were already so out of touch with your true self that you hadn't yet questioned the stories you were told growing up, that was me.

It takes a lot of courage to question the teachings of our past, our authority figures, our mentors, our parents, our grandparents, but when it comes to overcoming food, no rock, or stone can be left unturned, we must evaluate the values others have put on you, and the beliefs that others instilled in you. In the end, we keep what is truly useful to our personal DNA and we let go of that which no longer serves us.

You may investigate and keep that information, or you may decide it's not useful, and either way, you would be correct.

The People I know today who call themselves Christians are people I respect, and they always lead by great example.

They accept and never try to change a person, and they keep their judgment to themselves. They understand that growth comes for each person individually and there is nothing to force, time will tell its own story. Some transformations are faster than others.

Your judgment of others on God's behalf is unnecessary, in fact, according to Christianity, it's a mistake. And if you look up the word sin in Greek, it means a mistake. Personally, I don't believe in mistakes per se, I do believe we have experiences and hopefully, we learn from them.

We all have and will create experiences in our human state. Every time if the experience is not favorable it is our opportunity to grow. As a little child, I always knew when I was about to do something wrong, this intuition was there, it is built into my DNA, we learn not to trust ourselves through the restrictions of others, looking back I did that with my own children, don't touch this, don't do that, we lose our sense of self with every don't.

If only we really would have known to be patient and allow harmless exploration, we can't allow what we did not experience ourselves, we only pass on a vision for others that unfortunately is as limited to our own learning, values, and beliefs, we can change the world with changing this one thing.

The one thing is a limited vision for us and others, all things good should always be limitless.

I know what some of you are thinking, I would eat too many desserts.

Maybe you are confused about what is good, maybe your good or treats and beliefs about what is good are mistreating you, are your treats in alignment with your goal? Or are your treats mistreating you?

Since I didn't have a lot of adult guidance most of the time, this tells me I was born into knowing what was good and what was bad, I don't need someone to hammer it into me their way.

Especially their ideas and priorities for how I should or shouldn't live my life. If it bothers me consciously then it's probably not for me to do, but maybe consciously you may not be bothered by the things that bother me, then it's probably okay for you to do, you may change your mind later. When I grow in an area I change.

We must always know our own heart and mind, and the heart wants what it wants, and the mind is changing with every thought, in fact, we have something like sixty-thousand thoughts each day, and we don't even recognize the subconscious subliminal inborn messages from early childhood until we do, and that's where we learn and retrain our brain to the truth. Our own truth.

So many people go through their entire lives merely skimming the surface of who they are. Most never discover the profound truth and life treasures that lie hidden from a complacent gaze, to be revealed as a true lover of one's inner spirit and inner truth, and to be a diligent student of self-discovery.

Humans have lots of names for "God", I believe it is one source with many pathways and names, Buddha, Allah, God, The Universe, Absolute Spirit, Consciousness, Gaia, Jesus Christ, Divine Spirit, Holy Spirit, Divine Mystery, Divine Presence, Evolutionary Spirit, Great Consciousness, Great I AM, Higher Power, Highest Essence, Great Spirit, Man Above, Infinite One, Tao, Infinite Source, Lifeforce.

When I googled this, I discovered hundreds of names, all I know is it doesn't matter what you call it, it's there, and it's real, all acceptable.

When you are loving all forms of life, you are loving God, by whatever name you call it. That source is in you and will never leave you, you can call on it at any moment night, or day, It can do for you what you cannot do for yourself if you are willing to ask. You don't have to believe in anything, all you truly need is to just have the willingness to believe that it is possible that there is something out there is bigger than your compulsion, addiction, or anything else that is keeping you where you are instead of where you would like to be.

Today, I have a healthy respect for the church and church history. I am not tied to the belief that I must believe a certain way or do things a certain way for my soul to live on after it's done using this body. God did not do anything to me, or against me, God just exists, and I get to imagine this presence in my life in any way I desire. I do not believe there is a wrong way to believe in this thing that gives me life and breath.

IMPORTANT QUESTIONS TO ASK YOURSELF & Journal About:

What were you raised to believe? Do You still believe that?

Why or why not?

How does it make you feel to look at your belief? What would you like to believe?

What would you change or shift in your beliefs? What beliefs were forced on you by someone else? Are you angry at the person who forced it on you?

Are you angry at God? Why?

Is "the great spirit of life" Good or bad to you?

Why Good?

Why Bad?

What Do You Want this to be for you? Imagine "God" as it works for you, just for today. (There is no wrong answer.)

Now that you have your thought of who or what "God" is how does it feel?

CHAPTER 4

Broken Promises: We Stop Believing When No One Follows Through.

The inner self becomes what it is conditioned to become, it has no choice until it does.

When I was 6 years old, my dad went to Vietnam, which made my mother extremely happy. She wanted an allotment check and hearing her say she hoped my father would be killed, that he died, she hoped he got his ass shot, that he didn't come back, my mom hoped my dad died, oh, my gosh, she wanted my daddy to die!

As a little girl, I was so upset hearing this, I wasn't sure what death was, but I did know it couldn't be anything good, because my mother used her angry voice and then laughed in her usual cackle where my father was concerned, all I knew was that I was powerless and I didn't know what to do, I couldn't comprehend this in my young mind, it felt so heavy, it felt fat within me, it hurt me, the fear was like a tiger roaming its cage every single day after that, when the phone rang it was horrible, and when they were showing those draped coffins of dead service me on television, my mother and her children watched, to see if she could get the happy news that my daddy was dead. Walter Cronkite was not my friend. I was nervous about this, scared, and there was no one to tell and no one to comfort me. I was frozen in this feeling of powerlessness, it was like walking In deep mud, and my legs can't move because the mud is too heavy. Every day I waited scared of the news, every night after I was happy because his name was not there, and I believed if his name was not called then he would not be killed and would come home.

Finally, they stopped showing the dead men coming home on the six o'clock news, but I still worried I knew the truth of my mother's intention for my father's life. It was overheard.

Hearing my mother say that it was okay with her if someone was dead was bad enough, hearing her say she wanted my dad dead was another, it wasn't something I should have ever heard from my mother's lips, but I did I learned fear from my mom.

As a little kid I was doing this routine, wake up, worry, that today was the bad find out my dad was in one of those gray metal coffins, and then be relieved that today is not the day my dad died, going to sleep ver heard, hearing someone else's murderous intentions toward another's life in any situation is an out of line event in any situation, hearing it because of war tells way too much about their heartlessness and their intentions their negatively and as a result of it I never fully trusted my mother ever again, she could want to kill me, she sure didn't like me.

All she had to do was get a divorce, it's legal, it's acceptable, and no one should ever be required to stay in misery because of ritual or dogma, not that she was having any of that, but I guess hoping he was shot dead in Vietnam was cheaper than divorce lawyer which my grandfather paid for later anyway.

I was always caught up in what people were supposed to do based on those old bible teachings, and I knew thou shalt nots, even though looking back now I can see they are simply man's unreal expectations of himself. But she was serious as the day was long, and she gave the bad vibes if she was done with you.

Those men in the bible had a lot of wives, lovers, and concubines, they were biblical, right? Well, my parents were the same, I could identify with the stuff that was more like our house.

It was horrible to know that your mom was fine with your dad dying especially if he could get killed in some violent way that she approved of or thought he deserved, and worse yet I would stay awake sometimes at night and listen to her talking on the phone, mostly because she was so loud and her voice carried, or to her friend Naomi or Colleen in the kitchen, and I worried what she would do to me since she didn't like me either.

My Grandma and Grandpa who constantly rescued me from her hand were her parents, they were kind, gentle, and educated. I never could understand where she got her meanness, she complained about my father's abuses rightfully, I saw it, but she was mean too and bragged about what she could instigate and make happen.

I guess it is true, you can only see the things in others that you see, because you have them also. As an adult, I had to work on my anger toward her, which I took out on myself. Eating ½ loaves of bread, pounds of chopped ham, and dozens of cookies, but I didn't want to kill my mother, I didn't want to hurt her, but I did resent her for a long time, just like she resented so many people.

We all know things about ourselves we would rather not know, this awareness is a gift, because the awareness is what keeps us in check, and makes us more tolerable human beings in our society, our families, our communities, and our friendships, it is those who are clueless and living with no awareness of how they affect others, that we are in contact with that is the issue, it would be wonderful to pull a string and create awareness for others, unfortunately, we all must learn these hard lessons for ourselves.

We all learn at different times in life and a different pace, some of the people in my life will likely never learn and I will not have the pleasure of seeing change, others will, but I am long gone now so I won't know and either way it is fine.

I limit my time with people who 'bug' me, and I eliminate time with people who disturb my peace of mind, heart, soul, and who deliberately are mean and hurt me or disrespect me because I always believe those who tell me who they are through their actions and words. No going back to see if they can kick me again for this little lady.

The day before my dad was to ship out for Vietnam, my mother met him at the door with a sawed-off shotgun in hand.

He wanted to see his children, I am sure he thought or knew in his mind that very well could be the last time to see us, hug us, and hold onto us, she did everything she could to make us kids afraid of him, to discredit him as a father and human being, looking back at how she scared us, she was the monster, no doubt my father and her were in a physical war, but it must have been awful for him knowing there was always another man, she told us stories of her new boyfriends and how they were better than my dad, I remember one of them was a George, in my little world George was a curious little monkey, I thought she was funny talking about George, she justified everything for years, and then a wonderful thing called DNA became a part of our society, and yes she did have 5 children fathered by 3 different men while married to my father, infidelity really does cause knockdown, drag out fights, especially when a woman like my mother, gets in the face of a man like my father and brags about it, I wonder if my mom will ever know that some of her trouble was of her own making? Or more over that her trouble was her children's plight. It truly was a dangerous difficult and unfortunate situation for their children.

My mother didn't care about any of that, years later I learned my dad had carried us with him in his wallet, and his heart, and that is a comfort to me still today, it's good to know I was wanted somewhere. And that I was an international traveler there in his wallet.

I do know he set an intention, no matter how it worked out, he had never hurt me ever physically and I am sure my mother had great pleasure in denying him our presence and justifying his lack of parenting with her domestic abuse, but personally, you would hold a gun in my face once, and I would be out of there forever too.

I never ever blamed my dad for being self-preserving. But I did always want him to recue me and give me a horsey back ride again.

As an adult I know there are always two sides to every story, and I am sure men should not hit women, and visa-versa I like the idea of everyone being verbally and physically kind.

I also think that we could save ourselves a lot of tax dollars and money if the fighters were put in a cage until it was truly over, but then there is always that chance for change, and I wouldn't want anyone in the world to miss the opportunity, they can only do for themselves.

I remember the hitting going both ways, my mother bragging about breaking my father's jaw with a can opener, non-the-less she would not let us go with our dad, I wanted to go so badly, but she had the sawed-off shotgun and he left, I was always so afraid, a helpless little girl who cried, powerless, and I didn't know what to do.

Later, that same morning, my uncle Rex came to get us, he took us to grandma and grandpas house in Dumas, and my dad was there, I was happy, we were at Dumas, and dad colored in my coloring book with us at grandma's table, we ate, and I saw my dad, it was good.

Grandma took pictures of dad there with us that day, I still cherish those pictures, my dad in his uniform sitting coloring with his girls, (at least two of us were his) the truth was my mother wanted child support on all those kids, but she didn't want the ones that were his to see him or the ones who weren't his to see him, she wanted everything from everyone with nothing to reciprocate for anyone else.

I was just happy to be there at that moment, I really had no idea what a serious moment it was in my life, how necessary it was to make it a lasting memory, and of course, I wasn't afraid grandma and uncle Rex was there. It was fun. When mom and dad weren't together, it was fun.

Dad told me he was going somewhere, far away, (Vietnam) and he would be back sometime, and I waited, and waited, and waited, finally a long time after that I heard my mother say he was back and she could not believe someone couldn't shoot straight enough to "knock him off" and everyone missed him, they didn't have very good shots in Vietnam she said.

I was almost eight by then, and I was starting to put two and two together, and now I was starting to get mad and slightly confront her about these things, I learned again that she was mean. I learned to tuck my serious voice away and only talk about what they wanted to talk about, I learned to never share my true thoughts or feelings. I learned to be fake, put on a mask, and build a wall emotionally around myself, it was the only way I could be accepted, the one who lost was me, I survived but lost myself for quite a while. I forgot how to be funny and how to have fun.

I was so glad to know my dad made it back to the United States, he was home now. But I couldn't express it, now my mother was telling me to be careful my father might kidnap me. She kept me afraid and on alert with these stories.

Her stories of him made me afraid of him all over again, with the evil descriptions of who he was as a man and the things he would do if he "got me", she said bad things about my dad, but I was still glad he was alive and safe, even if she didn't like him.

Every day I waited, I wanted to see him, every time I saw a car like his car, my heart jumped, I thought today was the day my dad would come see me.

If I saw a car like his on the way home from school, I would sit on the front step waiting, I knew today He would come, I needed a drink of water but I wouldn't go in, I didn't want to miss him, If I needed the bathroom, I would wait, I didn't want to miss him, I couldn't even tell my mother what I was waiting for, I just waited, I knew he was going to show up, rescue me, hug me, save me, but he never did.

Those days of waiting were heartbreaking for me, and I couldn't tell a living soul what I was truly yearning for. He never did come; I didn't see him face to face for years after he returned from Viet Nam. All I knew was he did not keep his promise to come back to take care of me, he did not come back to me.

I was with grandpa once at the bank sometime after that, I was maybe 10, and my dad saw grandpa and even spoke to grandpa, but he didn't even look down and say hello to me, I was invisible to him I guess, a couple of weeks later he came to Dumas, I heard him early in the morning I was upstairs, I was so excited, he was gone before I could get downstairs, he was there, for them, not for me, he brought grandpa two snapping turtles for turtle soup, yuk, I was angry that I was nobody's child, I was so angry, I turned those big snapping turtles loose and watched them make a mad dash to the Des Moines River. It felt so good to rebel and it hurt so bad to know that I was not important to bother to make conversation with, to come to see or to be wanted.

I wasn't my mother's child either, I couldn't be myself around her, she was always having the next baby with the next man that she could lure, I never enjoyed hurting others. It didn't satisfy anything in me. As a little kid, I knew that hurting feelings and hearts was wrong.

How come my mom and dad didn't know that?

My grandmother tried to keep the peace and preserve the history for us kids, she would sneak a picture, or a glimpse of my father, when possible, when we drove by his house, I looked hard to get a glimpse, as anonymously as possible, just cars and a house, no dad.

If my mother saw a picture of my father she would destroy it right now, even if I was in it. It felt like she hated me too when she destroyed him.

Grandpa Laymon, my dad's dad, I remember him but didn't know him well, a big man in overalls, always friendly and happy, offered giggles and tickles, and smiles, and pink round mints from his overalls pocket had died, and mother said he died getting up in the night for a drink of water, and I better stay in bed, or I might die from a drink of water too, I believed her.

What she didn't tell me was he had a massive coronary. But mission accomplished, I was afraid to get up at night. I was a frightened 6+- year-old for no real reason, other than another way to scare me. It worked until it didn't.

They took us to the funeral parlor to see his body, he had his glasses in one hand and his pipe in another, the coffin he was in a big, long room with nice carpet, and people were standing around, I didn't know many of them, they were people my mom did not like!

I was six and a half years old, and I thought they must smoke and read wherever he was going off too, because he had his glasses in one hand and a corncob pipe in the other. I don't remember anyone talking about heaven or anything like that, no one told us anything about what happens when a spirit leaves this meat suit, we call a body and so what was I supposed to think about the end of life, so I had no way to know the meaning of the information.

Other than dead people were kind of scary at this point, they needed their glasses and could smoke their corncob pipe if they wanted to.

At some point, my biology took over and I went to the bathroom at nighttime, but that whole thing was just a cruel thing to do and speak. I remember saying something about that later in life and I was told I shouldn't be stupid and gullible, I was 6 almost 7 years of age, and my grandpa that I was not allowed to know had died. Humm, I thought.

Mother always says to me, seems to me like you don't like it here; I was always afraid of what she would do with me when she did decide to get rid of me, mom would always say, you don't trust me. Mom always gaslights me.

I guess that was true. Why would I? Today I can say that's probably true and totally okay. Trust is built on kindness and honesty, not mean intentions.

Everyone, my mother was mad at, she spent her time getting even with, at least in her conversations, but I wondered, you are here being mad, and they are there, and they can't even hear you talk these nasty conversations you're having about them, it seemed a waste of time, totally meaningless luggage to carry that no one else even knows about.

But I had resentment about her resentment that I didn't even realize for years, what do you do to get rid of that? I decided that you meditate and send her love, she doesn't have to know it, as a child I prayed she would change and be different, God didn't come to help me with her either, as an adult I send her love every day to this day, even though she did get rid of me some 48 years ago now, she still breathes, I do it for me. I did it for me, and I still do it for me.

I realized that I wanted for her and every other person who had ever hurt me, one simple thing, the things I wanted for myself, peace, and freedom.

I meditate today and send the universe love and all who are in it. I send hope for her and others, I don't know if they are open to receiving it, that's not part of my equation, mine is to send it. Mine is to be whole.

When we want good things for others, as good as what we want for ourselves that's when we reach ultimate health, when we can feel that love and send it to those who have hurt us unconditionally, that's when we are coming full circle, it's really wanting the same peace for others that you want for yourself.

My parents taught me a lot about useless efforts, I felt sorry for them, I learned quickly as a child if you don't touch the stove, you won't get burned, and they taught me not to cross them or expect anything from them at an early age, I became self-reliant at an early age, it is an awareness that grew with me, I eventually was ashamed of them for a time.

Then I realized I was ashamed of myself, not because I needed to be, but because life had put on me so much that I didn't know what was best for myself, my own life and relationships became sticky and messy, they were a mess, and because I wasn't taught how to get along and survive, I survived and coped the only way I knew how. Not the greatest, but glad for the ways it played out because I did survive!

I have learned to be grateful for the people who made my life hard, they helped me build an unshakable character that they interestingly enough don't like!

I became brutally honest at times with them. My anger eventually spilled out in my words toward them, and I was in this mental jail about them that I seemed to not know how to overcome, and I coped by eating compulsively, restricting food, and periodic binge eating.

Should is a word that should be removed from the dictionary, it implies you have knowledge that you have done something differently because you knew better, something you did not do that you knew to do. Or something you should not have or eat or be allowed to have because you have not used this unknown knowledge of knowing better than that in some way, or in some aspect because you did not use that knowledge had correctly in another's ideas, thoughts, or conditioning and now you are not enough, not good enough, valuable enough, please don't should on people.

Typically, when criticizing someone's actions, used on other people it is about shame, not being enough, don't go around shoulding on people, as if what you want has any value to them, if it doesn't, good for them, no one has the right to put should and shame into someone else's life.

No one else has the right to diagnose your life because you chose to live your life on your terms instead of theirs. Not one. Feel free to take your power back, do it diplomatically, but do it.

With age, I came to believe that my parents were clueless about the messages and wreckage they brought into the lives of their children, they did not realize that their actions, hurt or affected anyone else, but they did. Everyone's choices have cause and effect it simply does, for every action in this universe there is a reaction somewhere else, we are all tied together in this universe, body, mind, heart, and soul.

My mother and father finally divorced and by the time they did my mother had three children that were not my father's, she always bragged that up as though it was a pin in her hat that she could go off and have elicited sex and make another baby. With every baby she had, I felt further away from her. I knew I hated taking care of babies now. I knew I would never be good enough for her, I craved her love so much that I did things against my own conscious to please her. Then I was always ashamed because I knew better.

Birth control was available in the 1960s, but she was having none of that! She would have as many kids as she could and wanted to have been her statement to the suggestion, by grandma, and believe me she did.

It's probably a good thing she didn't take a precaution as it turned out she had a medical condition that would have maybe cost her, her life. Yes, I know she was hard to deal with, and no I never wanted her hurt, but sometimes as a child, I dreamed of her being in jail.

With each new baby, I was further from her in the line of kids. Pushed to the back burner, expected to fin for me, and take care of the baby stuff, I hated it, I knew very young having babies was not my goal, I didn't even like playing with dolls once I knew they were my having a baby training, no thank you!!

I was like every other child, I needed to be a child, I needed to play, read, have consistency, and even some responsibility, I didn't need to think of or worry about motherhood, I didn't need to have a baby to escape home, and I didn't need to learn how to do motherly chores yet. And maybe never, I did not want to be conditioned to the idea that the only thing I could be as a woman was a mother. There is so much more.

I daydreamed of being an artist, or an actress, a sharpshooter on a wagon train, a hippie chick, and Miss Kitty on Gunsmoke, she was so glamourous, and that was before I knew she was a madam and a hooker!

I thought I am going to see the world, make my mark, paint, teach, and have a career, I wanted it all and I wanted an education and to make my own money, and drive a nice car, and here I was seven or eight years old, I was cooking my own eggs for breakfast in second grade, and sometimes for my sisters. Being a mother wasn't on my bucket list.

My birthday met the deadline so I was put in school, I liked that, Aunt Mary and Uncle Rex were there, I got to see them every day, Uncle Rex would hold me up to the basketball hoop in the gym at our rural school so I could drop the ball in, we got two points every time, he was big and friendly and called me E-CHO and made me giggle.

Aunt Mary was slim and beautiful and always happy to see me. I was a little ragamuffin but glad to see them.

There were 42 kids in my 1st-grade class, I was lost, didn't know my ABCs, and couldn't count, I was lost due to the fact no one spent time in repetition so I could learn how to count or do my A-B-C's.

When I was at grandma's she read books to me, but it was occasionally. And if mom wasn't mad at her, not to mention mom didn't want grandma filling my head with anything, let alone a book, manners, or how to learn and be somebody, it was a great day for me if I was lucky and I got to be their kid for a long time like a weekend.

Grandpa would love me up reading the funny paper together on Sunday morning, I was a star a real celebrity at their house, I was in the funny paper, the best paper ever when you a kid. Tumbleweed's girlfriend was there, Echo was the little girl on the fence in that comic strip, and grandpa used to say, let's see what you're doing today. I felt special, little did I know-how on the fence I would be in this true world.

I really believed that the parents did not show up. Mostly because mine didn't, unkept promises trickled further than that and I learned not to trust, no matter what I earned by their standards, they never followed through, I didn't believe them anymore, they were never wrong or sorry, they lost my respect.

Every time I ever promised myself, I would do something, and I didn't do it, I was losing respect for myself, knocking my self-confidence to the ground, I didn't believe in myself anymore.

When I make an agreement with others, I make it with myself first. If I know the request is not one of my heart's desires or I don't have the time, I simply don't make the promise. It's okay to say no. The word no does not break hearts. Failure to follow through and keep your promises does.

IMPORTANT QUESTIONS TO ASK YOURSELF & Journal About:

Have you ever promised yourself you would do something, and you didn't follow through? Why do you think that is?

Did someone else make a promise to you that they didn't Keep?

How did you feel about yourself when this happened?

How did you feel about the other person when this happened? Did you ever say something you wished you could take back?

Have you ever promised to do something because you wanted to please someone else?

Do You still have the Disease Please? How does that affect your life?

Have you had trouble trusting people and realized later you didn't know why.

Do You Trust everyone, and then doubt that decision and want to back away?

What comes to mind when you think about this? (that's something to work on right away and be aware of).

CHAPTER 5 IDENTITY THEFT

You are confined only by the walls you build yourself - Unknown

Nothing of me is original, I am the combined effort of everyone I've ever known. Chuck Palahniuk

We moved away from that old brown house at Revere, where my mother used to lock me in the upstairs where the light was a window by the floor.

I remember going being sent to bed and there were still hours of daylight, I didn't go to sleep, I was just trapped in the attic room or whatever that room was called, the windows didn't open it was hot, it was summer, and it was dark when night finally came, I don't remember a bed in that room, I do remember a crib in that room, I remember my sister Crystal being in that crib, and I remember not being able to help her or get her out, I was maybe three years of age she was probably around ten months, and Melody must have been 2 and a half, we were there, for a long time, I was thirsty and dirty.

Sometimes when I am afraid my mouth still gets dry, it's not real though, I know that if I am having that reaction it is all about something I have told myself that likely isn't true at all, let me give you a for instance, recently my daughter put me in a group chat which included my biological mothers and my niece's phone numbers, it was near mother's day and as usual, I went down the line without looking at the group contents and wished everyone a happy mother's day. Harmless enough, right? You would think so.

My daughter went ballistic as though I was selling something to "her friends" with a Happy Mother's Day, but that was not all, she went further, she started making totally inappropriate statements in the group chat, and I cut her off at the moment, as I knew she was gaslighting me as she often does, I was bothered at first by her poorer than usual behavior, then I thought to myself, why are you bothered by this, you can wish anyone you want in the entire world happy mother's day, I thought about it, it was because she wanted me to look bad in front of my biological mother who had not been a part of my life due to her bad behavior, as though her poor treatment of me could be justified somehow when I realized it, I realized it had nothing to do with me, but the stories told to herself by herself or others, I went from hurt and embarrassed to relieved at the moment. The bottom line is it went back to old mom stories, I always wanted her to love me, but she never did, real love doesn't hurt and is not cruel.

Mom got a divorce from my father and a new man, he didn't like me, and I didn't like him, I was a kid, and he didn't even try, it was my way or the highway attitude with him. And of course, she was having another baby, this all met moving away, and grandma and grandpa were farther away, and it also met seeing them less, mom liked that, she didn't want them to know "her business" my parents taught me well the deceptiveness of their own humanity of every single thing that was a mandatory secret, if anything past a party of happiness and joy needs to be a secret in your life, I will be the first to tell you secrets are for the benefit of the mandatory secret maker, not the disempowered individual who is doomed to keep those secrets.

Secrets are your abuser's mandatory request, and as a child, you don't know what they will really do, or not do, but they have already done something hurtful or abusive or we wouldn't keep those secrets, we believe them because they already have. Our aggressors and abusers in your life, shame us into not telling the truth only to benefit and save face for themselves, it's their own shame that makes it need to be a secret. Not the abused, anything that needs to be a secret is potentially a problem, but mom had a new man, and off we went.

We moved to a little tiny house that had a gray sandpaper-like finish on the outside of it. It was 3 rooms, kitchen, living, one bedroom, and an outhouse out back. 5 kids and 2 adults, and we kids slept in the living room on the floor it was hard and cold, and eventually, we shared a bed in the living room.

My mom had a new husband now, he didn't like me, I told him he wasn't my dad, and he couldn't tell me what to do. He spanked me into hating him, and I did hate him, years later when he died it was fine with me, he was dead and it was fine with me, after years of being mistreated by him how could I be sad, even if he was dead.

He hit me hard on the head so hard it hit my teeth together and made my tongue bleed anytime I made the mistake of trusting him and getting too close, no child deserves that from any adult, discipline is needed with kids, abuse isn't. I remember crying so hard at his hand that no sound came out of me, the pain was so excruciating it had no voice.

He never talked to me again in a humane or kind way, which as a little kid made me sad, but also glad, but I was hiding out in life after that, not seen, not heard.

I learned how to be afraid the most from the people who were supposed to keep me safe. Life under that roof was hell and chaotic.

They eventually added a cement slab and 4 rooms on that house and put a couple of kids in each, and of course, no locks on the insides of the doors, only the outsides so they could lock us in as they felt it was needed if there would have ever been a fire, I wonder if they would have been accountable?

My mother was the true example of the law of attraction, you attract what you are. She looked for men with real problems so she could break them and change them, no one wanted to be changed by her, but she lathered it up thick about how awful their life would be without her, I am not so convinced that would be true, it was another man's disaster and man there was always another man, from this little girl's experience.

Worse yet I was expected to change my last name to the stepfather's name, my stepfather didn't ask for this it was a mother's insistence, and she was doing everything she could to get rid of any part of my father in her house, even his last name, my mother insisted on it, we were going to be a big happy family with the same name, I thought we had the same name, you didn't like it and got divorced and now I have to change my identity, I did not want his name and got whipped for saying so, I didn't want his name, mom made me, and I hated it, she told me when I go to school to write my stepfather's last name on my papers and that would legally change my name.

They may have physically forced me to change my name, however they could not change my mind, I would not give them that domain as a child, they could not change who I was in my heart, but they did make me feel of no value unless I changed my name, I hated the name, and I was ashamed of the name. I felt heartbroken to be forced into this against my will. My will was small. Now I just hated them for one more thing.

It legally changed nothing, it changed me, it took away who I believed I was, I was embarrassed and hurt by the demand, and I hated the name and the man, his people and family were mean, and I did not want them.

Now I felt stuck and how I felt about them was how I now felt about myself, and it hurt me, I didn't want to be the name of one of her men, I wanted to be my name, my dad's name, because it was my name, I hated her for that, she took away the things she gave me naturally, she taught me quickly how nothing was forever, nothing was real, just whatever she thought up for that day or week. she put my stepfather's name on my social security card, school records, everything, everything except my birth certificate, she couldn't change that without a judge, when I got a copy of my birth certificate, it had my real name on it I was thrilled! I was 21.

I jumped for joy actually, she had taken away every bit of my identity, I wore the clothes she wanted, I ate the food she put in front of me, I had no right to like or dislike anything, whatsoever what I was becoming was the prescription she made for me, the conditioning she gave me, and when I was twenty-one, I had the honor of untangling that mess of my identity for the United States government, the social security office, social services, school systems, and all other government agencies, she could do it, she could let other's beat me to it, but it was in no way legal!

At first at school, I did not put my stepfather's name on my papers at first. When I brought papers home with just my name Echo Laymon I got a spanking, mom said I wasn't even trying to be a family member, so after a bit of that I played her game and gave up who I was on paper anyway.

But I didn't like my mother much after that, she always caused problems with me myself, her underhanded dishonesty, just legal enough ways to get through life wasn't good enough for me, and my own values were bigger than my mother's even as a young child, I knew better than that.

The first day the teacher called me to the front and made me write my real name, on the blackboard 50 times, I told her my mom said I had to, it didn't matter. I was in trouble at home because I had to stay after and do the sentences when I told my mother why now the teacher was in trouble.

She called my mother and they got into a fight on the phone, my mother called her bad names and then called all the other parents and told them she was married to a black man, the next day none of the kids were allowed to talk to her because of that, I was hurt and so embarrassed, none-the-less, my mother won on all fronts.

The teacher resigned and someone else came, and worse yet it was all my fault for not wanting to change my name, I had the right to be me, my mom was the only person who didn't know it.

That was my first dealing with prejudice. I learned more about my parents through how they viewed other people than I probably wanted to know, I lost my name and all my friends all in one day, not to mention my own intuition and intelligence told me there is nothing wrong with any kind of people, no one can help who they are born to, or who their family is. I have spent my life from childhood trying not to in any way become a duplication of them.

What is wrong with my mom I thought? What was the purpose of doing this? As an adult I have come to realize that hurting people hurt other people, but that in no way makes it acceptable or excusable, it simply tends to hurt other people, and the people they drag through life with them, I know how important it is to realize that something is wrong in them, not with them.

I also totally grant permission to anyone who needs permission to walk away from toxic relationships and relationships that no longer are in alignment with your beliefs, I matured, and others never did.

As I type this, I look at my skin tone against this whiteboard and I am not white either. No one is. So, what difference does a person's skin make? What difference does it make how someone else chooses to live or chooses to live with, if they are not hurting themselves or someone else, funny my mother used to say that all the time, however, she was hurting someone, she was hurting me, her bad habits and bad blood hurt everyone she encountered, and she was clueless to that fact. Or at least that's the way it looked to me as the child looking up scared to death of what might or might not happen next.

We are taught as children to love everyone, right? But that was not modeled as truth by my parents, to each other, or to their children, it was a fictional illusion they satisfied and justified their own minds with, it wasn't what they did, So, now I saw no problem with interracial marriage in any situation.

I had learned so much at church from people who weren't even my people, every one of us is made by God, I was the sperm most attractive to the egg in the ovarian tube, others made it, but I was the strongest, with the strongest purpose, that's why I am here now. And I continued to push my way through a world of shit and came out on the other side.

David the guy who wrote the psalms, had 8 wives, and tons of kids, and killed Betheba's husband to get to her. Their son Solomon had over 700 wives and hundreds of children again. I liked it when they talked about the real stuff because I could relate as a child, I didn't relate to the perfect, un-messy stuff. The messes I related to. My parents were a mess. I felt like a mess because of the way my life was in their hands.

As a result of finding myself, who I am I took back my name, I was 32 the first time I wrote my name with no shame, no regret, and no guilt, Echo Laymon Pelster, I still use it today on my writings, websites, books, blogs, and identifying items.

My name is not who I am, it is something I have, and I choose to keep, it is mine, it has little to do with who I am, but today I know who I am, my name is mine and a part of my identity. And besides, I suspect if my mother is out there watching from a distance it really makes her angry, and honestly, that's the power she gives me in her cluelessness, and it feels like good karma.

Just another proof that we never have to do anything to get even, just wait, time takes care of everything.

QUESTIONS TO ASK YOURSELF & JOURNAL ABOUT:

Has anyone ever forced you to do anything against your will? What was it and how did it affect you?

Was it a battle of will that you could not win as a child with an adult?

If you could do it over again what if anything would you do differently?

What did you lose in the situation? Did You Gain anything?

Do you need to apologize to someone? Does Someone Need to apologize to you?

Did that person justify their position instead of apologizing? How did it affect how you saw yourself?

Are You Angry?

Is there Hurt and Pain? Can You let it go?

What if another person's opinion of you is not your true value?

How do you value yourself?

CHAPTER 6 LITTLE JOE

Trust cannot live in the same space as secrets and lies.

If you want to keep a secret, you must hide it from yourself--Unknown

By age nine, and third grade I pretty much knew that I was in control of absolutely nothing, and there was nothing I could do about it.

On this unusually warm December day in 1969 mother had told me to feed my brother Joe, it was oatmeal and totally a lumpy gag a maggot morning, with warm cow's milk straight out of the cow.

You might say I wasn't Goldie Locks, and I didn't like my porridge, and I didn't, I was always sick to my stomach with any kind of grain, and no one was paying attention to that.

I didn't get to pick what I liked; I don't even remember ever in my childhood being asked what I would prefer. It would have been like a dream for someone to ask me what I would like, or what color, or what kind, it just wasn't a reality for me as a child, I didn't know that other people were allowed to make choices about simple things, it still amazes me a bit.

When I shopped with Grandma and stayed all night with her I always got to pick, what cereal I would like for breakfast, what color of new blouse, and so on, at home it was dictated for me.

As an adult, I do have preferences and it is not rude to ask for what

I would like to have, the color I would like to wear, anything, but it was a long time coming because I was truly never asked or given choices, so I pretty much took what was offered up in my life, even the plates of bullshit, because I did not know I could choose, other people did choose, and the sky did not fall when they did. The world did not run out of anything as a result, and there still remains plenty of everything, everywhere, for everyone.

Learning not to wait for the approval based on limitations of others thinking and beliefs, choosing to think for myself would become one of my greatest assets, it was the one thing I could choose to do in any situation. I no longer follow a lead cow in life, I think for myself.

On this December morning, 1969 I had sneaked and thrown my oatmeal away in the backyard that day because, if I didn't eat it, more than likely it would be in my place come supper time all dried, soured, and crusted over and I would not get anything else to eat until I gagged it down and maybe even threw it up again. I learned to be deceptive to not have to ingest what I did not approve of for my own body at an early age, I know it was probably wrong, but it was what I could control, so I did.

If I did eat it I would probably throw up on the way to school on the bus and get sent home, at the time I was an undiagnosed celiac, and lactose intolerant, we just didn't know that then, and I wouldn't get anything else to eat until I did, the food war had already started between me and my mother by then, she constantly told me I was a fat slob like my dad.

I believed I was very worthless because she made it so adamantly clear, that I was the first pancake, the throwaway child. She just didn't understand why I didn't just go away forever; I finally did. To this day I am still gone. I offered her a chance to change the end of her and I's story, she refused, and I felt free. It is what it is.

My dad was not fat, at least not then, and neither was I but her messages made me see my body in a distorted way at an early age, and the angry words, did well for giving me self-doubt, I started looking in the mirror seeing myself as fat, as a number, not as a person, I wanted her to love me, I wanted her to care, I tried so hard to please her, and of course, I never pleased enough. Looking back at old pictures I was not fat; my mother was not accurate. My little young mind believed her. Something can be a lie and you can totally believe it, at least until you sort it out and know better.

If I, did it the way I was told to, it wasn't good enough, and if I didn't, it wasn't good enough, I learned there was no pleasing her, and if she wanted something, really lookout because there was an even bigger price to pay. Mostly I learned to disappear and not try.

Anytime I was in the presence of my mother, and she was being kind to me, she either wanted something, or she wanted to know something she thought I knew or wanted me to do something, it was never just to spend time and be happy and content with me, the whole thing made me an anxious child and adult for several years until I was able to identify these behaviors in myself and others, I could always feel my mother's physical deceptiveness, that's the empath part of me, but as a child, I couldn't identify what I was feeling so much, and feelings were neither acceptable nor necessary in our house I felt everything and had to sort it out later in life. Feelings are a part of our DNA they are happening every second of our life, even in our dreams. They are very necessary.

I don't even think she knew or was aware of how she was seen by myself or others. Her idea of life and how it was in her own reality seemed to be the life of all who stayed nearby.

My daydreams as a child were about leaving and going far, far away. To be a writer, artist, and to sing, I made the mistake of saying that out loud in more than one family arena, to be told I needed to be something that I could support myself with, so I listened to everything everyone said, did the job everyone thought I should do, and I was miserable for years. With each job change, I found a niche or pleasure, finally getting me back to here, where I truly wanted to be. In a way what they pulled me away from gave me a story to write, their neglect and abuse from my perception became my largest asset. I wonder if there could have been an easier softer way to get to here from there. Probably, but I have an amazing strength because of all of it and I am grateful for that.

I am sure it was not the intention of those family members that I would ever do or be anything to anyone, but that's ok, from where I sit it feels like more than just surviving, it feels like thriving, and you can too!

I grew up and went somewhere else and I had the same problems in a different place because I had not yet figured out that I had to change my own mind, I had to change the conditioning I received as a child, I had to take responsibility to the best of my knowledge, here and now. I had to integrate the job I had with the job I wanted. I had to transition my entire life and make it mine.

I had to change what I could now and wait for what I couldn't always watch for opportunities, and not be too hard on myself in the process. When I saw an opportunity, I took the risk and completed it quickly. My advice is not to ponder things too much, to have faith, and leap when opportunity knocks. Sometimes I would leap and think what the hell, catching my wings and inspirational airflow on the way down, and every time I was better off than where I started.

Because every time I had the courage to try something new, I was already a winner, I love to embrace change.

Just because an adult says something does not make it true. It is not who you are, and it is not always your personal identity. You are the light and essence of God's presence embrace that light.

The I AM lives deep inside you, your mind, your heart, and spirit, the ultimate love, joy, and kindness of the self within. I had to have it for myself first before I could give it to anyone else. It's not something I owe anyone, it's something that is earned through mutual respect.

My brother, Little Joe didn't want to eat his oatmeal either, that December morning, he cried, he said I hate you, and I told him I hate you too. I offered him another bite and he said I hate you, and I said I hate you too, again, that very day he was hit by a train and killed before I came home from school, I felt ashamed for the things I had said that morning, I was trying to cope with myself and my awful words, while rumors flew about in whispers of why this three-year-old was near the railroad tracks unattended, suddenly our family was becoming a pariah, and I was never able to take those words back or say I was sorry.

I could confess to no one as I knew I would be blamed further as he was supposedly chasing my beloved beagle Buckey when the train hit him.

My life suddenly became more complicated, more complicated than losing my name and my identity publicly, now people were asking where my mother was, I knew sometimes when I was sick at night she was not there, so I wondered about the answers that day and knew it might be true from my own memory and experiences of waking up in the night and going to mothers room, and no one is there.

I kept the secret of that conversation to myself for many years, I hated that I saw the truth of it in myself, sure I realize now that it is the kind of things kids say to one another, however, it was locked up and pushed down inside me, frozen in time, no parental guidance to re-examine the words, we were never taught how to be nice to one another, mother mostly played us against one another, something that went on then and still does.

In the past years I have stopped by my sister's homes, and they don't answer the door, they need approval I guess to live their life their way, I grew up and away and took control of my life, it saddens me to watch, I know I did nothing wrong, except one thing. I broke away from the dysfunction and chose to own and take responsibility for my life.

It had a cost, the cost was great, but I chose correctly because I am not hostage to the craziness of dysfunctional game playing, manipulation, or attitudes today.

I didn't tell grandma because she was always saying honey, be careful with your words, I didn't tell my mom because she would just use it against me every time anything came up, like so many other things, the God I was raised with sent you to hell, so I was silent about it. I just didn't ever tell anyone I hated them ever. I chose my words much more wisely; I learned the irony of regret by age nine.

I realize today that all of it was only an experience of what you might not want to do or say, but you might also, but until I could get grown up and had a bit of insight, and an understanding of the conditioning I was raised with that put the whole idea of my own wretchedness into my subconscious I could only believe it, not change it, and the way I handled that old conditioning was, I pushed it down with cake, mistreated myself with treats that mistreated my body, and other self-damning activities.

Today, I know with all my heart what we see wrong in others is what we need to work on in ourselves. We attract what we are, and those who don't like what you become will sometimes leave your life instead of accepting your new internal intelligence and intuition for your life.

When I chose to stand up and not participate in the hurtful mindset of my family, I was simply rejected by them, hooray! It did not feel like that at first, however, I had to figure the hooray out for myself, the good news for you is you can stay miserable trying to change people to be who you need them to be, or you can change yourself now! I vote for the latter if they ever make a change that is built and bound in truth and significant change they will seek you out, in the meantime, you can choose to be the best you, you can be, and live happily that is your true birthright. It has nothing to do with who you were born to, or where you live.

I call that voice, God's voice within me, it leads me home, in my evolution of growth every time I listen. And it's hard work. Awareness will do that to you.

Worse yet every time mother told a story of what happened the day that Little Joe was killed it was different, so we kids didn't really believe her after a while. The last time I asked her she said she didn't remember, I wished I didn't.

I was nine years old, and I believed my mother was a liar, I dared to say something twice and got belted across the face for questioning her, with a do as I say, not as I do comment, I wasn't cured of how I thought of her, but I did learn to keep it to myself.

The day little Joe was killed, Aunt Betty came to get us after school, which was weird, as she lived up the road by and never did come to get us for any reason before or since that till that December day.

Once at her house she wanted us to hide in the bedroom underneath the bed, it was so odd, to go to someone's house and hide under a bed, we wondered what was going on, it didn't make sense.

I realize now they did not want us kids looking out the window and maybe seeing an ambulance or a police car, or the removal of my brother's body, we would have been asking questions, questions no one knew the answer to, looking back I can see that it was the wrong kind of protection, to protect us from the truth and then abuse us with the answers when the questions were finally allowed to be asked.

Then my mother's second husband's father came to get us kids from Aunt Betty's trailer house, and said, you kids need to go home cause Jody is dead, I said Jody? Who's Jody? He slapped me across the face and said that's your brother, and I said no, my brother is little Joe, I think back to that moment, and I can still smell the chewing tobacco and cow manure on that old mean son of a bitch of a man, again mother had brought another horrible man into our lives that later would hit us with a bull's whip, spit his chewing tobacco on the floor, tracked cow manure all around the house, and if you wanted to eat at their house you had to wash your dish first. Eventually, that Bull's Whip got lost when he left it unattended, we were resourceful self-preserving children when we found an opportunity. It burned well.

Once we were back at our house, crying and upset and not understanding, having lots of questions, and not being allowed to ask them, we kids sat and whispered. Our own stories were our reality.

No one told us anything, we were just supposed to know what death was and understand. Mother came in and got an outfit for Joe to wear, a Red Barron sweatshirt, Jeans, and boots. I remember thinking you need clean clothes when you die. If you are sleeping forever, don't you need pajamas? She had an angry look on her face, we were stifled and quiet.

When Kids are left to themselves they make up their own stories about what is happening every time, and when we become adults in fascinating families like mine, we must rethink everything we were ever told or thought about, to make a life for ourselves takes a lot of courage, and I was tenacious not to mention downright stubborn, I knew there was more for me, and the heart wants what the heart wants. I wanted to leave and go as far away as I could get. Love was never the issue; it was the crazy things that drove me away.

Every story had to be reexamined and every value put on me re-evaluated, was it a value for my life or a value someone else had that I was expected to live by?

I was the only one who could find out. I was the only one who could claim my own answers. No one else can know what is best for our life, we must do that for ourselves.

Guilt is not a spiritual technology that has a purpose or serves anyone, we are all a part of the heart of the infinite life power which I chose to call God.

All powerful and limitless. Whatever thee puts in my heart and mind I can hold in my hand, it is thy truest wish for me.

Even as a little kid and you are not sure where it is you are driven to go, I knew I was unique, special, and gifted, I don't know how I knew but I knew, and I just always knew I was going to go. And

I was going big because I wasn't going home.

Since no one told us anything about dying, so we just had to think about it on our own as little kids, we were marched up to our brother's casket and looked at poor dead Little Joe, dead, he did not look like how I remembered him two days earlier, in this dead stillness it was as though his face had changed, as children we did not go to the funeral, and we did not understand that when the life spirit leaves the body so does the color leave the skin, the sparkle of life was still alive, just somewhere else now. No one told me that I decided that had to be the way it happened later.

So, we stayed home with a babysitter when they buried Little Joe, and people brought us cake. Lots of cake. I thought it was strange bringing all this food over to have a party or celebrate like Thanksgiving Day at grandma's or Christmas.

As a child I was hurt, no one was telling us anything, or asking us anything, no one even wondered about us, it was like we were invisible in the middle of a herd of people and a hundred cakes.

I had my feelings so hurt from the other step-grandfather's whack across the face, my insides felt as though they were jumping and shaking, I could feel the sobs inside that would not come out, the fear inside me was pure devastation and everyone was worried about arranging the cakes and finding enough table space, the dead little boy and they had no concern for the living children, four girls, age nine and under that day.

It was awful. We kids were clueless about protocol, death, its meaning, and its consequences.

When I finally had the courage to approach my mother about what happened to Joe, and what it meant to be dead, what she said exactly was, "what difference does it make to you, you never liked him anyway", and now she was telling me how I felt. So I did not ask anymore.

I never asked anyone again, but I and my friend Joyce walked 7 miles at 9 years old to find the cemetery where he was. We walked down the highway to find out because I needed to know something, anything.

We got in big trouble for that, we were just curious, we just wanted to know. I wanted to see this grave, I wanted to know. My heart wanted to see and know.

People just kept bringing cake. I remember lemon cake; it was amazing and when I ate it, I felt better inside. Every bite of those desserts and cakes made the hurt inside my heart go away.

I could eat and not get full. Those cakes were my first official binge I think, my first true connection with food and medicine to fix my heart and as love, mostly because no one was loving on me when things were awful, like that. But no one was loving me when they were good times either.

Grandma always tried, but mom resisted, we were her pawns to be used as needed where grandma was concerned. Grandma talked bad about mom and mom talked bad about grandma, it was best to just talk about something silly or nothing when you were a little kid.

After that anytime I was anxious, hurting, uncomfortable, unhappy, or afraid I instinctively knew to reach for cake and other sugary foods, and they always neutralized how I felt, of course, this was unconscious until I had conscious awareness of it, a mouth full of rotting teeth, and a first conscious decision that I was going to not eat like that anymore, I could not stop I would try, I didn't know why I couldn't stop eating sugar and then I started learning about it and other white substances and it all made perfect sense.

Sugar is 30+ times more addictive than cocaine or heroin, I totally know that today, sugar is noteworthy as a substance that releases opioids and dopamine and thus might be expected to have addictive potential, (nebi.nim.NIH.gov) it's just like any other craving, if you starve it, it goes away if you feed it your body wants more and more, eventually you cannot take in enough to feel better, it no longer worked like it once did, and calm can't be found in the sugar fix, and it gets bigger and bigger, and so did I.

Two things have been true for me in this life, two things have been proven to never be retrieved, first is my words, once they are out of my mouth, their tone and honesty are forever heard, by someone in some way, I have learned to think about what I am saying and who I am saying it to, I can say what I need to say stay true to my values, even though I can apologize if I am aware and you live long enough. Words cannot be retrieved.

The other non-retrievable in this life is time, On the day of Joe's death, I learned that I am not the master of time. I chose to live today in the best possible model and opportunity to not regret my own choices, I am not 100%, one hundred percent of the time, but today I chose to think things through to the best of my ability. I learned regret is a heavy burden. Once a moment is spent it cannot be retrieved and spent again.

QUESTIONS TO ASK YOURSELF AND JOURNAL ABOUT:

Has anyone close to you left or passed away and left you with regret?

What is your regret? How Can you fix it now?

Do you cover up your pain by eating? What do you eat?

Have you been forced to eat foods you don't like?

How do you rebel?

Are you making all your own choices of foods today?

Are you still rebelling with your food choices and behaviors? How does it serve you?

Do you have unanswered questions from childhood? Can you get them answered now?

Would DNA testing get clarification for you? Are you afraid to find out something?

What?

What is the worst thing that can happen?

What creative thing can you do yourself to resolve the question you have?

Would public records help you?

CHAPTER 7

The Murder of Bucky

An eye for an eye only leads to more blindness.
Margaret Atwood

Two days after Little Joe's funeral I came home to find my dog Bucky dead, my mother said that her husband, my stepfather killed him because little Joe chased him, and that caused Joe to be by the railroad tracks, the rumor was that my mom wasn't even home, but to justify the circumstance of this three-year-old's death, to make it more palatable, their answer was to murder my dog Bucky, my beagle had to die too, Bucky was dead, his spirit was gone, his tail wagged no more, my heart was broken, broken more than when Little Joe was killed last week, why didn't my stepfather blame my mother, she was supposed to take care of my brother, but they killed my dog, Bucky's little beagle body looked in pain. I was silenced and muted out of fear, and I knew I could not say anything to change this awful event.

My mother's 2nd husband my stepfather fed him a raw hamburger with glass crushed into it, she said, and they left him there for me to see, and yes, I got the message, I lived with monsters, I lived in fear, and I was angry, I wanted to do something, anything, but I was little and afraid, even at age nine I knew I could not overpower them so I learned to push down my anger, out of that fear, the fear was real and necessary because my parents were unreasonable and mean, the actions of my parents, proved I must be self- preserving,

I must protect myself, I pushed away the hurt with food.

I would go out looking in ditches to find pop bottles to turn in for the return deposit to get money to buy candy, I was like a drug addict trying to get his fix, only I was a little kid trying to get to sugar to feel better.

And I could not get enough food to relieve my pain. I realize today what I was feeling was anxiety, I never needed drugs for this once I knew what it was, my drug of choice was sugar, once I knew its identity, and I understood how it worked, I only needed to change what I was taught to believe about myself, once I did that my weight started going in the other direction.

Everything I felt about my parents, and other people who had hurt me emotionally, physically, or financially, everything I felt toward them I took out on myself. They didn't even know how I felt, I was too ashamed to admit I had feelings about anything, after all anytime I did I was pushed down, beat up, or insulted and ridiculed to such a state of shame that I had to stay in hiding from society itself.

Hindsight is 20/20 I punished the wrong person, Me!

I unconsciously aimed and fired at myself, coping with them.

I believed I was defenseless at the time. I kept their horrors to myself. I kept my anger to myself because I believed it was not acceptable to be angry, I should have broken the family rule about telling family secrets by telling someone. But the secret, it was a secret, and secrets cannot be fixed. Secrets can only be unveiled and the stories we tell ourselves about those secrets must be rethought and unraveled.

We had it screamed into us as children that we don't tell family secrets at school, we don't tell grandma, or we won't see grandma, we were scared into believing the welfare people would come to get us and take us away and we would never see our mother again forever, looking back perhaps more of us could have survived, but we were kids, and we were scared.

In every crowd there is an abuser, a victim, and a bystander, I hope if you see something going on, even if it's only a suspicion, that will have long-term effects on another person's life, that you will step up in love, caring and kindness, it will be the most courageous thing you do in your life, regret weighs much heavier than the risk of insulting someone.

The secrets and lies at our house after Joe's death only escalated, my mother had another baby on April 1, 1970, since she was pregnant with number 6 when Joe died. That was the year she got a new boyfriend and became a truck driver, running steel for a junk man to Peoria Illinois, she bragged how they loaded the steel with lead and got paid top dollar ripping people off.

Apparently, this man had lost his CDL license for violations undisclosed to me as a child. My mother was so proud of her smartness to wear a mini dress and go-go boots to deliver the criminal steel.

She bragged about how they would schnook the buyers at the big steel yards and made out like bandits. I was a little kid and I did not think it was cool, I was ashamed of what they were saying and I did not want anyone to know what my mother was a part of, she would tell you those were her days of working for the mafia, she was so proud of that Idea, I think The Godfather movie inspired this I suspect, these people had no connection and they were not a connection anyone with any sense wanted to make.

I was 10 by now and not as dumb as my mother would like me to be. I knew my mom was not anyone important to anyone of value in her relationships, those men used her more than she used them, she always gathered people around her that she believed she was smarter than, it was her way to look smarter to others, and control those below her on the food chain mentality, and if she looked that way to me, I knew other adults ought to know too, unfortunately, it was still a time when people felt they should mind their own business, which is good, but not when harm is being done, I have learned a lot about the blind eye in my lifetime, there is an abuser, a victim, and a bystander in every group gathering, unfortunately, I do believe all abuse should have intervention today, an obligation to report, and taking a mind your own business attitude allows millions of children and adults to be sexually abused, tunes a blind-eye to domestic violence, and especially emotional and physical acts against children, mentally challenged adults and the elderly.

I know from my own experience no matter what my mom did, I still loved her, that's what kids do, mostly because they are hostages without any say. Abuse whether emotional or physical is more comfortable than the unknown scary places you have been warned about.

I loved her because she sent me to religious institutions that told me I had to love her and forgive her, why did I need to love her, if a so-called classmate or friend treated me bad she wasn't a friend because she didn't act as a friend acts toward a friend by her choice of how she treated others, but in families, the family gets to stay family when they hurt others, they get to be loved unconditionally anyway, that's messed up thinking.

Forgive them for yourself, so you can be free, but realize you owe them nothing. I choose to give grace for my own freedom, I don't put myself in harm's way out of ritual family expectations or even reunions anymore. I no longer hear the voices of shame in my head that my mother placed so gracefully and probably more cluelessly than I gave her credit for.

I believe in forgiveness for those who say they are sorry and admit their wrongdoing, they admit their abuse and violations of others, and they are living a life of change, not manipulation to make themselves feel better in the moment, how do you know right, you don't, humans are humans, we will always make some experiences worse than they need to be, but when we become aware of the fact that we are in control of our responses to every event in our life, life changes, life's outcome changes.

I don't believe in handing out forgiveness as if it is confetti, I do believe we attract who we are, if it keeps happening we need to look at ourselves and our part in the events of our life and past, unasked for or requested forgiveness given automatically breeds an attitude of come one come all, you can come to do that to me again, anytime you want. I do believe in giving open forgiveness and grace to those who are by their own admission both sorry and wrong.

Yes, I do believe in accepting apologies if you are so inclined, it does not mean I trust you, this person unconditionally, or owe them anything, it means that your side of the street between you is cleared, and it doesn't mean that you need to invite them back into your life, that's the choice of each person for their situation.

Forgiveness is good for your soul, I believe that it is freeing morally and spiritually, for yourself if, for no other reason, you can forgive anyone, you don't even have to tell the person if you don't want to if you are ever supposed to tell them, I think you will intuitively know that you are needing that connection for that moment in your life, but it is not a requirement. Sometimes we forgive someone in our heart and mind, and suddenly they reach out to us, the universe responds for you in this, it's up to you whether you pick up the phone should it ring.

Either way, it is okay, but not mandatory by any means, every situation has two ingredients in it. Sometimes we don't even remember what someone else is apologizing for, that's their level of consciousness, some people will never apologize for what we think they should apologize for, that's our level of consciousness, I am not sure either is incorrect.

What you do with the information in your personal decision-making is totally up to you. In all situations, there is amazing room for the humanity of mankind to step up, free themselves, and free others, it's a choice we each get to make.

I also know that just because you apologize about anything that does not mean that the other person will ever accept your apology, you apologize for yourself in the right opportunity to do so, please know you cannot control or predict the outcome, your value is not reflected by the opinion or acceptance of the apology or your words, you can only control yourself and your intention, in the good and healing of a relationship, just don't be attached to the outcome, the outcome and response of the person you apologize to does not even play into your self-worth and well-being, if you are sincere you have done your part, move on, enjoy the freedom of doing the right thing, getting the past out of your head, re-writing your future and how you will act or re-act toward others because of the experience. You have a new learning curve and a valuable lesson.

I only have the power of knowing and understanding my own intentions. Never others.

QUESTIONS TO ASK YOURSELF AND JOURNAL ABOUT:

Has anyone in your life ever been cruel to you or another living thing around you?

Was it punishment for something else that happened that wasn't really your fault? What happened? How did You react?

How did you handle the anger?

Did you think there was something wrong with you because of their actions?

Did the action of another person cause a loss of life? If so, how did you deal with that?

How did how you dealt with it change it? What would you do differently if you could?

Do you feel guilty about anything?

Were you blamed for something you never did? What is something you did to get food?

Did it change what happened in any way? Did you get in trouble if you cried as a child?

Where you insulted or ridiculed if you showed emotion? Were you told to shut up? Suck it up? Or stop balling?

What would happen if you screamed right now? How did it feel?

How is you hunger after screaming? (In an appropriate place of course.)

What do you think will happen if you let out what you feel instead of pushing it down?

Who have you had a million conversations within your head that you need to tell off? Write it out. (It's yours for no one else). Say what needs to be said.

How does it feel to get it out of your head and on paper?

What other parts of my story can you identify with. Write it down.

CHAPTER 8

Alleged Right of a Parent

Any alleged "right" of one person Which necessitates the violation of the rights of another person isn't and can't be a right"- Ayn Rand

When I was 11 my mother took me to planned parenthood to get an IUD. I remember she made me and my sister where dresses that day, I remember the doctor questioning my mother about why she wanted me to have this, I was a virgin, I did not even know what being a virgin was, or meant, I did not understand, and it didn't matter if mother said you have to do it you did, I felt violated and I hated her for that, she had no right, she did not own my body and she could not make me like the men she introduced me to that were her age, I heard the doctor say my sister wasn't a virgin, I didn't know what it meant then but I do now, and what the hell was going on that my mother thought it was okay to get little girls dates and birth control against their will?

I understand why regulation and law have gotten into the family business today because not all families treat their children like family. I also recognize that many of the people who fight certain laws around the exploitation of children are the ones breaking those laws.

I knew this junk man should not be "lying down" with my mom when my other stepfather was at work, this was not because he was tired, and of course, if he was why was my mother lying down with him, wouldn't he sleep better without someone bothering him? Even if it was in my mother and stepfather's bed?

He was always there. The stepfather went to work on the three to eleven shift at the iron ore plant, and just like clockwork here he came, coward of a man, he had a wife at home, but I am sure from what I saw of him she was happy anytime he was not around, He was mean, and he was unpredictable, by age ten, I expected nothing less of my mother.

I had never even been interested in a boy, in fact, my body at that point looked more like a boy.

When I told grandma about things at home, I got in trouble. Grandma didn't get to see us, for quite a while, that was the punishment for all of us if we didn't mind their own business, the long stretches of not seeing grandma was hard, it was the only time I felt anyone cared about me sometimes, mostly because others were working or away, so I learned not to say some things to grandma, or at least feel things out with her and then decide if I could tell her, after that grandma and I had talks and I didn't tell mom, it kept me safe.

I learned the difference between keeping secrets, what happens to you by an abuser is to benefit the abuser, and keeping confidences, which is having a private conversation, telling your truth, and sorting it out a bit, a practical way to process information and find viable solutions even as a child, we always have a choice in how we react to our circumstances, I told what happened and stayed with grandma pretty much every chance I got. To this day I have never understood my mother's sexual manipulation of her children or grandchildren. It's a sick ticket I don't understand.

I remember thinking maybe it's not just us. Maybe everyone's mom acts like my mom. Maybe everybody's mom pulls your teeth out with plyers when their tooth is rotting and they have a toothache, it made my toothache worse, by the way, my mom never had the money for anything I wanted as a child, she had the money for coffee and cigarettes and nice dresses for her to wear for her boyfriends, but not for kid stuff, I think she pulled my tooth so she didn't have to spend her cigarette money on a dentist, and maybe everybody else's mom gives their kids mean ugly haircuts and nearly cuts off their ear doing so when they are mad, but I know they didn't because other kids made fun of my hair, my clothes and my family, I knew my mother made our clothes because it was the cheaper way, it would have been nice to get to pick out the pattern and the fabric. That wasn't the case for me.

I remember saving nine dollars of my own money to go to a real beauty parlor and get a permanent wave, I loved it, my mom didn't, she just started cutting, my brand-new hairdo! Now it was ugly, I learned don't do anything that is not Mother's idea, because she won't like it and you will pay by being ugly for the next several months while growing it out.

I remember wanting a pretty dress like one of the other kids and the answer I got was that's not practical, and you don't really want that. I really did want that, it seemed like anything I wanted, any feeling I had, that was not in alignment with the adult plan was always denied.

But I did want, and they were wrong I did want pretty things. My wants were never important to anyone except me. I really believed I was not worthy to have nice things or have the ability to be more well off, most of that was the meek shall inherit the earth, really, I thought, those who work will have what they want I learned to work, I am still working I hope I never stop working. Work has gotten me many things that I wanted.

There could have been a kinder understanding, but there wasn't, so what I wanted didn't matter unless somehow my wants benefited someone else, it didn't so I didn't get a store-bought dress.

Mother would convince me later that I did not want something like a new dress, store-bought, by telling me how fat I was and how unattractive it would be to my slobby figure. I believed her, she got her way, it worked.

I should cover up my fat don't show it off. But if she made me one of her homemade dresses from her hookers or us selection, I was expected to wear it and like it.

I realized as an adult that I was raised with a myriad of double standards that always benefited someone else. I had to learn as an adult what I preferred as clothing because truthfully everything was imprinted by someone else's idea of who I should be and what I should look like. The first time I tried on an outfit in a store that I truly liked I was truly uncomfortable.

Maybe everyone else's dad left too, and their mothers had other husbands and boyfriends and a new baby almost every year, maybe everyone else's dad beat their mom, and never even came back to ever see their children, I cannot believe as an adult what was acceptable and forgivable under our so-called Christian roof! Christian my hind end!

Jesus, I imagine never intended to be justification for and forgiveness of the intentional bad acts of humanity, or maybe they had 50 stinking guinea pigs in the kitchen and cats that shit anywhere in the house, and maybe they are embarrassed by the childish behavior of my mother, maybe I can run away from home and find out the world is better elsewhere. I daydreamed about going somewhere else, anywhere else.

I wouldn't let the forgiveness clause of Christianity ever become the crutch that made the bad acts of my parents justifiable, that forced beliefs down my throat, that they didn't do themselves, they justified their divorce of one person's adultery only to become the victim of the next husband or wife that did the same thing, holding the silence and the secrets of their vile crimes against their children and one another.

The Religious Christian forgiveness clause kept them out of jail is what it did, those rules kept their children's victims and helped them and their egos over justify their humanity.

I forgive them for their ego, that overlooked my emotional needs as a child, and I celebrate my consciousness of all that has been revealed as a result of passing through them, I celebrate the resilience of spirit that I hold as my own eternal light today, the resilience I have beheld because of my experiences of passing through their lives.

I celebrate the spiritual consciousness that I hold with God in my soul, the light revealed that no matter how I felt, I was and am never alone, I will not allow myself to be entangled in religious beliefs that hide the vilest crimes under such an archaic guise, a belief of hell and damnation does not have the power to set any spirit free to live in its true calling. I forgive them for being them, I do it for me. Whatever their God does to them is between them and God. But I choose to not accept judgment and condemnation.

As a child, I worried something was wrong with me, however, once I escaped my mother's household, and self-destructive lifestyle, I realized it wasn't about me, it never had been, but I was still doing some needless suffering, I was holding on to the resentment, I couldn't trust others even though they had done nothing wrong, It was because I had become what I was, I attracted what I became, and my life was showing, it was all an illusion, but it was my illusion.

I had to find a way to overcome all the experience, hang on to the values that mattered, which turned out to be grandma and grandpa's values, and throw away what wasn't and hadn't worked. If an idea does not serve me any longer, I let it go.

The anger at my mother hadn't worked so I stopped being angry, I meditated and sent her love, praying for the enemy became pure bliss. After a while the anger was gone, through the process, I realigned the process of who I was with who I wanted to be, the truth was I had only wanted for my mother first and then my parents what I wanted for myself.

I became a person of influence, very good at sales, teaching, and learning, I chose not to live my life through the rearview mirror, but through the windshield of life. And not looking back at what I could never change gave me a freedom that I had never experienced and allowed me to master my emotions and not be the instant victim of someone else's opinion.

Besides, opinions are like assholes, some of them are bigger than others and some stink more. Don't know who said it first but they are absolutely right.

I often say to myself, you are healthy, you are healing, you are healed, thank you, please forgive me, I love you, and sometimes I say I am sorry if I realize something new, but I do not apologize over and over, as my soul has a good memory, its where God lives, and God does not forget my request and holds nothing against those who apologize for the negative things they become as a result of life's experiences. God is the light within, the light of the life I live, celebrated, and accepted, a consciousness of love, joy, and kindness.

Whatever your abuser accuses you of is what they are likely doing themselves. Whenever they discount your feelings, undermine your desires and opinions, or try to tell you something is different than what you are seeing and experiencing they are gaslighting you, emotional sabotage to try to make themselves look right through your eyes, they are often narcissistic and, they can't be outwitted, they are best left alone, just as you would a rattlesnake. Even if they are family sometimes it's best to just move on out of harm's way.

I can only change myself, you can only change yourself, those they' s can only change themselves, it is not our obligation or even our business to think we need to work that out for anyone, convince anyone, we can't, so we should not have it as a goal or a task.

As we take care of our own business and focus on ourselves with self-love and self-value, we cannot be embarrassed by the actions of others who do things to shock others, these people are really only amusing themselves with your misery, they enjoy other people's pain, they love the sting of their shock.

Mom didn't want to be known, her business was always to be her own, So, I guess my mother's boyfriends and bedfellows were a secret, but how? It was okay to know about them but not talk about them.

The cars were parked in front of our house in a little town of 400 people and 500 dogs, and God only knows how many cats, and then there were the 50+ rodent's my mother kept stinking up the kitchen.

Everyone knew she was not keeping her promises to her husband except for her, to her, every decision was justifiable and excusable, there was always an excuse or reason, if there wasn't she would make up a whopper with lots of shock value just to make sure, she was the only one who was clueless, everybody else knew what was going on.

Sometimes people asked questions and made snide remarks, I was embarrassed I didn't know what to say, I truly wanted to hide.

I learned that anything that needs to be a secret except a surprise birthday party or another loving awesome event, is toxic waste, if someone is trying to silence you, embarrass you, or threaten you, this is what they are protecting themselves from.

Upright honest relationships do not ask you to keep secrets, they are kind and loving with lots of appreciation and celebration in them. They do not threaten you with hell or evil, they hold you up to the light, no light can ever be found in dark acts or negative fear- based threats and actions, you are a light, never allow someone else to put out your light for their own benefit.

Secrets keep you in the darkness and despair, Openness, Honesty, Love, and Integrity always hold you in the light. Find a light and share the secrets.

QUESTIONS TO ASK YOURSELF AND JOURNAL ABOUT:

Has a parent or other adult forced you to do anything with your body against your will?

What did they threaten you with? What is the story as you remember it? Do you think your memory is right?

Have you been told not to tell or keep a secret by an adult?

How did that secret benefit that adult? How did that secret hurt you?

Are You still afraid? What still scares you?

Knowing that fear is F-ALSE E-VIDENCE A-PPEARING R-EAL how can you walk through your fear today.

CHAPTER 9

Shot and Raped

"Man is not what he thinks he is, he is what he hides"

-Andre' Malraux

My mother took a defensive attitude when questioned by her current husband her second husband, my first stepfather, who suspected the next baby born in 1974 might not be his, she was, but it was just an obvious violation of his trust for her, she always tried to make him believe he had an over re-acting with his imagination, she tried to make him believe he was crazy and she would do no such thing, he was on target. In 1974 I was 14, and yes it was obvious to everyone who could see the truth. It wasn't papa bear hanging out in mama bear's bed.

1974 was a horrible year, I learned the power of other people in other ways I had not known before, it was May 13, and I was about thirteen and a half at the time, I was just starting to like boys, but I had no way to judge a good or bad boy, I was never taught anything about the opposite sex except the adult examples I saw as role models. Looking back wasn't a role model at all, but long story short, a boy paid attention to me, and I thought it was cool because he was older than me, I was wrong, I was a young girl and someone to prey on.

He was not the handsome knight in shining armor that other young girls would ever dream of. But as a young girl, I had run out of dreams, I was uncomfortable with my body, and my looks,

I now believed every bad thing my mother and others ever said about me, I didn't have low self-esteem, and I had no self-esteem, and because I didn't, I was easy prey to anyone with selfish self-serving intentions.

That day this boy came over, he sat in the yard at our house with me and acted like we were great friends, some of my school friends kept driving by, I wondered why all of a sudden because they never did before, but I was naïve and always gave everyone the benefit of the doubt back then, little did I know he had told everyone he was coming over to make me, I didn't even know what that met.

My mother came out in the yard, and he asked her if I could walk him home, she instantly said yes, I wasn't even asked I was just expected to go because she gave permission, something did not feel right to me, but I went, once at his house, he gave me a slug bug bruise on my arm that hurt so bad it brought me to tears, I turned around to go home and he told me he was sorry. Come in and he would get some ice for it right away, again I was naïve, there was no one else there, it felt all wrong, I started to leave, he grabbed me, and he raped and sodomized me.

When it was over, he made it out to be a love affair, I wasn't talking, I was so hurt and angry, he insisted on walking me back home, he told me how I could have been his girlfriend if I could have had sex better! We didn't have sex! He had sex, I had never had sex before, and I did not have sex that day, I was raped and he was a creep! How would I know the expectation? It was awful, during the rape, he bit me.

I was in a lot of pain, I made the mistake of telling my mother, she told me that it was what you could expect from men, I was never married to a man that acted like that later in life, so I guess mom was the loser magnet. I never trusted her again; she should have at least asked me if I wanted to go. She didn't, I felt like she set me up, she was always trying to get me with a guy. Because he was a boy more than one of the older men, she was always suggesting for me I was caught off guard. Sadly, she was glad I was finally broken in.

Two days later he came to our front door, he wanted to talk to me I must have scared the shit out of him, he told me that if I ever told anyone else, he would kill me, so basically, he and my mother had to have had a conversation because I hadn't told another soul. Every day after school, I had to watch out because his stepbrothers and buddies would shoot me with their Beebe guns, I became afraid to be at my mother's house, now I sought out the idea of staying at grandma's all the time, I knew I couldn't tell grandma if I did she might do or say something, and if I couldn't stay with her it would be worse.

I was running scared, and I couldn't tell a soul. I was bitten by another human with no medical care, and I didn't know what to do, I was so trapped. It had nothing to do with me, I don't believe anyone ever attracts the bad acts of another human being, we all have to be accountable for the things we do to ourselves and others we have no accountability for the actions of others bad or good.

I was manipulated into a bad situation that I didn't see coming because I was a needy lonely girl, due to the absence of parenting and neglect. Statistics today show that children like me have a risk 90% higher than I did in 1974, so basically neglect your kids and they are at risk. I didn't know that until 2021, it explains how it left my own daughter generationally dysfunctional in this area also, I couldn't teach what I wasn't taught, we cannot do better till we know better, and that is no one's fault. Life truly does happen.

My mother had eight children with 5 different fathers, which has turned out to be the awesomeness of DNA, the truth again can be revealed!

My mother thought DNA was wonderful because men couldn't get away with not supporting babies that were theirs, the other side of the coin, women could no longer accuse not-guilty man. It works both ways.

When I was 14 my stepfather #1 after my dad, of course, filed for divorce and divorced my mother, I was 14 by now, and my mother could not stand him leaving her, and staying at her best friend's house, he went to live with one of my mother's only friends since childhood, she frothed at the mouth about this, how dare her friend take him in, they must be sleeping together, she had to have him back, she got him back, she married him again.

QUESTIONS TO ASK YOURSELF AND JOURNAL ABOUT:

Have you ever been sexually violated?

If not were you threatened somehow, sexually? Did you tell?

If not, how did your rapist create fear in you? Are you still afraid?

Why?

Are you ready to take your power back?

If you could do anything in the world to that person to make them pay, what would it be?

Write it out use your imagination, I am granting you permission to get even on paper, dear diary it.

How did if feel to grant yourself permission?

CHAPTER 10

Stepfather's Death in My Playhouse!

The most painful goodbyes are the ones that are never said and never explained - unknown

When I was fifteen, the stepfather supposedly killed himself in our playhouse, although my mother told me to lie to the sheriff and say exactly what she wanted me to say that day, she told me that she and her junkman boyfriend, had killed him, as she said the words, she told me, not a gesture, a suggestion, or a hint, she said the exact words.

I was shocked, scared and frozen in that moment, I was like a puppet, it was as if I could not think about anything that was happening around me, it was horrible to know, horrible to know I was supposed to say something that wasn't true for her when any other time I would have gotten in trouble for lying, but lying for her benefit was okay.

Believe me when your mother tells you something like I just killed your stepfather with my boyfriend from the junkyard you don't know what to do, but your automatic caution light comes on and you are working mentally in fight and flight mode.

I kicked into survival mode, the mode, that was the most in alignment that supports my life, survival mode, I thought in my head if this little 5'2" woman who weighed 130 pounds could kill even with the help of this man who was 6'3' man who weighed 205 pounds or so, who often crushed my head with his fist that was as big as a cantaloupe, I trusted that she could and would get rid of me if I didn't cooperate, scared to death I lied to the Sherriff. I told the sheriff word for word what she had instructed me to say.

I knew I would drown in the Mississippi river if I didn't. I haven't swum in a natural water source since. What I knew about death at that very moment was I did not want to experience it that day or soon after.

The stepfather paid a hell of a price for coming back to her, but to protect the boyfriend he needed time for him to get into a bar fight and get thrown in jail so he would have an alibi at the time the body was found, so he went to Illinois and got arrested. June the 15th. 1976 was a hell of a day in my life. Or should I say hell day?

My mother's friend knew there was something wrong with the whole story, I saw a letter she had written to my mother accusing my mother of her husband's murder.

After the funeral of the stepfather anytime we walked into a store or church or did anything in public, the room was suddenly quiet on our arrival, it was embarrassing and awful, to say the least, and my mother would say things like I am not going to let them run me out of anywhere, they're just a bunch of jealous old bags.

They're jealous of someone's husband suddenly dying, who is found hanging in their neighbor's children's playhouse? Who? Who is jealous of that, that is what was being gossiped about.

The whispers of all the suspicious behaviors, comings, goings, gossip, and rumors, were unbearable, I had stopped going anywhere I did not have to go, I was becoming more isolated in other areas, and I was already hiding out from my rapist and his posse, and now I had to hide from people I had known my whole life, even the church people where my mother insisted on sending us to our whole childhood, suddenly no one was ever going back, mom was burning bridges for everyone in the house, we had ever known, it would be years before I reached out on Facebook, again, we were gone overnight, without explanation, it was traumatic and extremely scary.

The Junkman boyfriend was around a while after that funeral, but he seemed self-preserving and moved out of the picture. If they were seeing each other, it was no longer obvious, he was gone, and she was on the next manhunt.

Later mother came up with a story about her being a mafia bookkeeper, and he was her enforcer, but now he had released her from the obligation of keeping the mob's books like they're going to let someone walk away who supposedly holds so much information in their head. Some more of her crazy stuff.

If they were all in the mafia, I would like to know why we lived in a squaller and eat beans and macaroni for our diet. Had homemade clothes and no shoes sometimes, hardly any power or wealth and pride, and we weren't Catholic either.

They must not have been very smart mafia people; they drove junk and were broke all the time. I would say they were want-to-be gangsters.

The Godfather movie Part II came out that year, I think she adopted it as her next story, the story that would justify everything. I was under the thumb of others' stories and Someone else made me do it.

My mother was crazy that day making us kids wait in the car, going back to the house not letting us get out of that 1970 Toyota Corolla, it was a hot day in June, I and my 4 little sisters were in that car, (one sister had a job, so she wasn't with us), mother would go back to the house, leaving again, going back, why are we doing this?

Mother would say, I am trying to get him committed again he wants to kill himself, which was a farce, I am sure looking back it was an alibi excuse, a rumor of justification, her idea of self-preservation was to make her husband look and sound suicidal, to throw suspicion off of herself.

Bessel Van Der Kolk, M.D. wrote extensively on this in the book The Body Keeps Score, my body kept score on these events until I released them through police reports and told the true stories of what happened that June 15, 1976 day.

Finally that day she left Kahoka that day, for the final time, and she dropped me off at work, I was so relieved to get out of that car, I needed to pee, and I was hungry so I could get food at the restaurant where I worked, I had a horrible feeling in my gut, I knew something was wrong, I could feel the lies brewing, I was right, but I could have not known how right I had been, I had no idea how right I was till later that day.

About a ½ hour later our neighbor showed up to tell me that my stepfather was dead, and I needed to go home with her, again hindsight was 20/20.

Had I not gone home with her, my mother could not have forced me to lie, and I would have just told the truth about everything that day totally cluelessly, and maybe not lived with so much anguish about the lies I told to protect my mother who hated me, threw me away with lies and deceit, and has never picked up the phone or called me personally in 48 years, she hated me then and still does. Her freedom did have a price it was me. The unwanted pancake child. No great loss I am sure.

The lie I told on my mother's behalf that day was that her husband, my first stepfather who made the mistake of marrying her twice had been acting strange all day, that was the lie, I can't tell you anything about what that man was doing that day, because I never even saw him that day, dead or alive, not that day or the day before.

When I awoke that morning mom herded us all to the car where we stayed in that little red 1970 Toyota Corolla from 8 am approximately to 4 pm in the afternoon, back and forth, through every single trip back to the house, even when we returned once, then twice, and then a third time, she forbid us, kids, to get out of the car, she would not let us get a drink of water.

My mother would leave the car, go in the house when we went home, and into the courthouse, stand in the hall, and talk to people walking by in the halls, she was not going to an office, my mother was creating her alibis with every conversation. It was the only explanation that the latter made since.

On one trip back to the house to sit again in the car in our driveway, I could see the junkyard boyfriend's pickup was in the back yard by that shed, we could see the truck when we left again for the third time, and we weren't allowed to go into our own house even to go to the bathroom, not that day.

I was scared to death that day they found his body and hearing the words come out of my mother's mouth, she admitted to helping kill her husband, and the idea that she could do something like this, little did I know that me being a parrot for her, and saying exactly word for word verbatim as instructed, would keep me under investigation for years, that old sheriff in Clark County Missouri was not as dumb as my mother would like to believe in 2017 I finally gave up the ghost and did a formal report.

When she said she could take care of me or get rid of me in the river I believed her, I believed her because she always hung out with people from the bottom of the food chain, with no manners, no education, no money, and very little moral turpitude.

That old Sheriff told me he knew I had nothing to do with it when he pulled me over with a speeding ticket at age nineteen.

He told me all he wanted me to do was tell him the truth, and I truly wanted to, however, I was more afraid of my mother and her friends than I was of the Sheriff, I did believe my mother when she told me as long as I was quiet and didn't admit to anything no one would ever know. Well, I was quiet, and no one ever did go to jail. But someone did know, I knew.

After My stepfather's funeral and the whole ordeal, she said that her boyfriend the Junkman killed him, more than once, then "she didn't really help", I didn't believe her, she only helped hang him up with his belt, then mother started telling new various other stories about him drinking brake fluid, and then it was something else. I guess she was trying to change the rumors concerning this dead man.

Eventually, she stopped talking about it, she was getting some hate mail, and rightly so. Her only friend totally and completely abandoned her at that point, you know the one that was sleeping with the stepfather supposedly when he left her that time. I could understand why people chose to escape our family through distance, it was the best thing for those who could escape, I called those the justification stories, "he was going to hurt himself" her justification stories, it was like hearing it was okay because he wanted to die anyway. She was extra crazy during the summer of 1976.

My mother allowed my sister to keep the belt he supposedly hung himself with, not sure whatever happened to that family heirloom!

It gave me the creeps to see it laying around our bedroom. Every time I saw that noose in our room I was sidelined into thinking about escaping.

Yep, you heard right he supposedly killed himself in the kid's play shed, so thoughtless, I thought over the years. Just another great childhood memory! Thanks, mom!

I kept her secrets even after she betrayed me, I still protected her crime against me.

But people were not as fooled as she would like to think, she was not as smart as she thought I suffered from horrible anxiety, and I was afraid of being arrested me being a 15-year-old kid who regretted lying to the Sheriff, it was years later before I realized they don't arrest people for lying unless its perjury in a courtroom.

But she held it over my head and tried to make me look incompetent all to save her skin, I realize a person can only be found competent not incompetent, that was another error within my mother's threats against me, the more educated I became as an adult, the more I realized how she played with words to manipulate her victims.

She kept us as ignorant as she could so we would believe everything she told us because we had nothing to weigh it against, no education or real facts.

This was the year I found the book Blood Letters and Bad Men in the library it was very interesting; I saw traits of my mother all over that book, psychosis yes, gangster no!

I finally did file an official Sheriff's report and told the truth and total timeline of that day June 15, 1976, there was only one sheriff's deputy still alive, but he remembered the case, I felt better, and I knew if they ever exhumed that body the truth would come out. I am sure from the stories she told he was poisoned somehow and hung up after he was dead.

When I finally made those full police reports in Clark County Missouri, because I could no longer keep mothers' secrets, and filed the report in 2017, in early 1980 out of fear I had written my first book and copywritten it in 1981 to protect the information and the timeline.

I knew without writing it down it would be lost in subconscious memory, I believed she was telling it differently to confuse us on the remembered facts and the stories she was telling, she was clever but not smart.

I spent years being absolutely horrified that somehow, I would be implicated in my mother's crimes and life events, and not remember the exact facts to protect myself, my mother had such a way of trying to brainwash me, and on paper, now I couldn't keep from telling the truth any longer, I had to get it out of me on paper, tucked away, copy written, in a safe place, in the safe deposit box.

I knew over the years that if something was wrong with my mother's story that day with my mother and her behavior, she never would have forcefully asked me to lie, she wasn't worried about the little kids that day, she could control them, I was an older teenager and I was asking questions already. She had to dismantle me and discredit my credibility quickly, or I might let the cat out of the bag. She did. Fear is a powerful antidote.

And let's face it you grow up and realize you don't want to be loved by the monsters of your past; you don't need to apologize for that either.

I permitted myself to not need my mother's love as a condition for my survival and success. I decided to blaze another trail, a trail of love, hope, and joy for others who suffered from traumatic parents.

I am living proof that no matter how devastating your life has been, no matter what has happened to you, no matter what has been done to you, and no matter what you have done to yourself you have the power while you cope with it, you can overcome it.

When my mother remarried so quickly to a man she met through a letter, the dead stepfather's cousin, she married him 2 days later, sold our home pulled up stakes, and burned all bridges, never even told our grandparents she was taking us out of the state, we were gone without a trace within days literally uprooted.

I was my mother's biggest problem I knew the truth, and I wanted to go home, I wanted to go back and live with grandma, and I wanted to tell the truth.

Within 10 days of arriving in Nebraska, being in a new school, and keeping big secrets, my mother signed me over to the State of Nebraska as an unwanted child. She made it seem at first like I had some kind of mental defect, I was unruly, and in trouble, however, the authorities blew a hole in her story pretty quickly when they checked with our prior town authorities, my former school where I hadn't even been in trouble, except for smoking in the girl's bathroom, which was not a crime, just breaking a school rule, the more they visited with me the more they assured me that they knew nothing was wrong with me, but I still wasn't talking, the only thing I asked is since she doesn't want me to do I have to go back there since I am not really bad.

They said they would find a place for me. I went into foster care until I was emancipated, and I never went back to my mother's house for a single night ever.

I thought I would be allowed to go back to grandma and grandpa; however, mother covered that base, she discredited them also, that way I couldn't get to the people I trusted the most. It was almost a year before that process was over, and of course, they had no record of any kind, no violations in life except the deception of my narcissistic mother.

I was picked up at school that day with the clothes on my back, I never ever had my personal childhood belongings returned to me, I rarely saw my sisters ever over the years as they were either killed or dead, or brainwashed by our mother about me, I never spent a night in my mother's house ever again, and when I went home I went to grandma's the only place that ever felt like home and safety really anyway.

What my mother intended to be hard for me turned out to be the most awesome gift, at first being thrown away was painful and left me broken-hearted, however every day I seemed to find something amazing in my life that deep down would never have been available at "our house" with each gift I became grateful for being tossed away.

During my childhood, my mother always told me that if you talked to the law or a psychiatrist they would shoot you up with Thorazine and other truth serum and then lock you away forever, so I didn't talk to anyone I was sent to for my well-being in foster care because I believed my mother, I just tried to be nice because her memories were my first weapon of defense, even if they were mean and ugly I couldn't risk trusting anyone she taught me not to trust.

QUESTIONS TO ASK YOURSELF & JOURNAL ABOUT:

Has an adult ever asked you to lie for them or keep a secret? What was the lie?

How did it make you feel?

How did you deal with lying or protecting an adult who did something wrong?

How did you feel about the adult afterwards? Do you trust this person?

How has this person tried to discount your intellectual property and make you believe there is something wrong with you, not them?

What did they say to make you doubt the event and how you remembered it happening?

How did they justify their actions later?

How did you feel about yourself because of their manipulation? Do you manipulate others to justify your own manipulation?

If you could do it over again, what would you do instead? Was it worth whatever they promised?

Did they use it against you later? How did it create fear?

Write a bit about this event in your journal or diary. It's just for you, say what you need to say.

CHAPTER 11:

Given to Strangers

I am no bird: and no net ensnares me: I am a free human being with an independent will

– Charlotte Bronte

The only real prison is fear. And the only real freedom is the freedom from fear.

-Aung San Suu Kyi

My every need was always met, and I was learning new skills and possibilities every day.

During the fall weeks of 1976, I seemed to be remembering 1972, I was 11 almost 12, when Secretariat won the triple crown, I remembered and missed grandma and grandpa all the time, I missed the good times at Dumas, and I remembered the weekends we watched Secretariat run the Kentucky Derby, the Preakness, and the Belmont by over 30 lengths, I remember how we jumped up and down and celebrated, I remember how we told aunt Mary when she arrived later that day, we had so many good times there, riding the horse, and fixing food, giggling, and just being ourselves. It was the place I could always be myself.

I was in foster care, sick and overwhelmed by the fact that I thought I might be pregnant because I had never ever had a period I didn't know for sure, but I thought I could be, the night before we left Missouri I sneaked out of the house I was going to run away to

Dumas, to grandma and grandpa and tell them what was going on, I knew they did not know that mom was going to take us away and we were never going to see them ever again if she had her way.

That night I went out the back road, and there was a huge bonfire by the slough, there was a guy there that I liked, and I decided what's the hurry, so I hung out, and then we hung out, but it was my choice and as it turned out I was pregnant.

After we arrived in Nebraska I was sick, I was in the hospital, in Lexington, which got me away from my mother a lot, the doctor kept asking if I could be pregnant, but I kept saying no because I didn't think I could be, I thought you had to have a period to have the ability to have a baby, I finally had one after I had a child.

I was 16 when my son was born.

I was 15, traumatized looking for love in all the wrong places you might say, and pregnant, and I was sick every time I ate pancakes or smelled certain foods.

I was sent to an unwed mother's home in Omaha, and I intended to give the child up for adoption, being a parent was never a part of my personal plan. But I was going to be one whether I planned it or not.

I had nothing, I didn't have any money there, I was washing my clothes out in the shower and drying them in the bathroom at night or hanging them in a closet on a hanger, I used a bar of soap, I got by.

I was provided a bed, desk, shared bathroom, and bedding, and 3 meals each day, we went to school on site, and the nuns and priests held chapel meetings, I told them I couldn't have an abortion in the foster home because I was Catholic, now I told a real lie that was my own, I think it was in the line of who I would recreate myself to be, my third husband was a cradle Catholic and I joined the church when I married him. In fact, the priest that married us and blessed our life passed away on June 4, 2022, we will be married 25 years in July, which goes to show you get the right priest it works.

I felt it was the right thing to give the child up for adoption, I was barely 16, life had been hard, and I didn't have a full education or a way to take care of him, but I knew I could love him best by giving him up, then my mother reared her ugly head, with nasty phone calls, threatening me that if I gave the baby up she would adopt it, it happened back then, she didn't want me but she wanted my baby? So, I kept him because I knew he would be hostage to her and bait to keep me in line forever. She was still running my life.

Now a parent I was emancipated, 16 years of age, and living by myself in a town where I knew no one, back in Lexington I went to school and my child went to daycare, I had to live in a house my mother and her newest husband had purchased, I was back under that thumb, I hated my life and felt like I had no choice in life. It was my fault because I didn't tell or fight back, and I chose to have sex with a boy I liked. So, my life is what I am attracted to now.

Mother always had babies, but I had never wanted to know anything about them, I liked my sisters I just didn't like their poop and spit up, remember it was not part of my plan, so I was learning the hard way. He had colic and cried a lot. And this time it was my fault. And my own child's diapers and spit weren't as bad as others, so I did have some maternal unplanned instinct.

His days and nights were mixed up and he was hungry all the time. I started him on cereal so he could rest sometimes and not be hungry when he was 3 days old which is unheard of these days.

I was sixteen I did not want to nurse a baby, I had watched my mom use her plopping a boob out anywhere and anytime it suited her to shock someone or empress she had jugs on a man that was nearby, my sources were limited for this little boy, I fed him two parts carnation canned milk to one part water. It was what I could afford, and he survived, I made about one hundred dollars a month so I could afford some of what we needed.

I had a crib and a bed in that house, a four-burner gas stove and a coffee pot, one pan to cook in, and a refrigerator that worked most of the time. I shared a bedroom with my baby, and the sofa was on the floor.

My mother and I really didn't have anything to say to one another, we kind of avoided each other mostly, we didn't talk about what she had done, what she had done to me, basically, the attitude was nothing had happened, I knew I wanted to see my family and sisters it was important to me, the few visits I had were horrific and terrifying, eventually, she moved back to Missouri, left me in Nebraska, and I didn't go back except to see grandma and grandpa.

I just stayed away, especially after she told me, don't you get it I never want to see you again, I was loyal to her and in return she shunned me. The secret keeper never wins, secrets can't be fixed.

I discovered that trials were some of the best defining moments in my life, trials helped me change behaviors that got me into the places I didn't want to be, like if you don't want babies don't have sex without birth control. If you don't want to be in debt, don't spend more than you earn. Date longer so you can truly get to know someone before you get married. Learning how to move through the crisis in my life was not as simple.

I wanted to see my sisters but since I was only two blocks away, they would come over, and sometimes they would babysit for me so I could walk after groceries. I got a job after school for a few hours and they would babysit after daycare closed till I got there for an hour or so, I didn't have teenage life, I went to school but was made fun of because I had a baby, or boys would say rude things, so I didn't ever go to ball games, or other school events, just school so I could feed my baby something better than canned milk.

At this point, my mother hadn't spoken to me for the better part of four decades, except for slightly cordial family situations such as funerals that could hardly be avoided, a few holidays for an hour or so, we just don't mesh, it's her choice I choose to honor her wish, I have peace and serenity when she is not in my life. I used to hope to re-write our story to a happy ending, I let it go a long time ago, I really just wanted others to know they are not alone, and in reality, being dumped as a child turned out to be the best thing that ever happened to me.

The statement I gave the Clark County Sherriff Office was about freeing me, not convicting her, (although my sister's father died, and they lived a life without their dad while she received a nice monthly check.) It was about freeing me; I was in a jail without bars. I knew that even in a murder case if there had been too much time more than likely the cold-case file and trail would be hard to follow, I had investigated the laws and statutes, but I needed to free myself.

The statement was a decision that freed me from my mother, her behavior, and her past which I was pulled into simply because I was her child, I decided to encounter the fear, stop the guilt, free myself, and take back my own power through the statement, what the authorities did or didn't do as a result was not my business or my problem, it was there's I had release the truth. It wasn't mine anymore.

I AM Free from worrying about the other shoe dropping in the future. So, I did it. And my anxiety that I had carried for 40 years was cured almost overnight. I guess that church stuff was right, the truth will set you free. Which by the way is old ancient writing before it ever made it into the bible! There is nothing new under the sun.

Until life at home with my mother, wasn't a secret I realized I could not be free and live well completely. It wasn't what I was eating; it was what was eating me!

I knew that if I went through with a statement, all the chaos could unravel way beyond what I imagined the worst could be. No matter what was happening in my life, that day was always in the background.

When I gave the statement, I was fully able to forgive her, because I didn't have to carry a lie that was not mine any longer. Carrying the lie, being forced to say something I couldn't even respond to with choice in such awful circumstances was in the same realm as being raped because I did not have a choice, I was engrossed in an extremely traumatic situation, I walked in the house and mother grabbed me on the spot, the sheriff walked in the door within seconds of the instance, I had no time to think, no ability to react, fear had me in a place where I could not feel as though I could breathe, no chance to make a choice, no chance to decide if I should lie for my mother, she always told us lying would get us in more trouble than telling the truth, she was right, her lie sucked at my soul for years, I have never had trouble taking responsibility for the things I did or didn't do, but the burden of my mother's lie on June 15, 1976, stirred my life with fears, problems anxieties, and trust issues, what happened that day happened in a few minutes and changed my lifetime, in a very few minutes.

Since I had discovered sugar was a powerful good girls' drug, I had been trying to find an easier softer way, sugar was my drug, and I coped with sugar. I unconsciously ate every memory repeatedly until I had gained weight clear up to 357.8 pounds. I was diagnosed with congestive heart failure and pulmonary hypertension at age 37. I wanted to live, and I was willing to go to any length to make sure I did, even if it meant telling the truth and facing the consequences.

Today I haven't eaten sugar unconsciously for years, because of all of this, the cycle of my own life, I have developed a coaching program to help other people who hide in obesity and food addiction, that are still struggling to find their solutions, and live their values. Me going public helps others find me as a resource for private healing and responsible coaching skills.

As you can see something good does come out of the most horrible things, after 2 horrible marriages the first one didn't work because it was my mother's idea, see I was pregnant with my second child at 17, I did not marry her father either, he thought I should have an abortion, I just couldn't do that, so I married to have my baby, bad decision, good baby, after being alone for several years figuring things out, learning, and knowing I could financially take care of myself. I will be the first person to say pregnancy is not a reason to marry anyone.

Figuring out that I am very smart, I met my husband of 25 years this year at my sister's funeral, after her suicide about a year later we started dating and then married, look for the good, there is always bad in the bad, see that the creator does provide and does align, sometimes we just must look harder and sift through the circumstance that makes us feel a lot of bad emotions and feelings to realize the greater purpose in a circumstance.

We cannot get to the glorious moments in life by going around the trials, we must walk thru the burning coals sometimes to get to the peaceful nothingness and feel the existence of God within ourselves.

Right there within me, not something to be sought in the mist, the spirit is here, it's here for everyone, however, we must acknowledge it as our light to activate it with acceptance and faith to preserve the knowledge of and practice the presence that the existence is always there, there is no doctrine, no right thing to wear. Come as you are. Just bring yourself.

As each of my mother's husbands died, we saw this pattern, and each time we rolled our eyes and knew we were not hearing any kind of truth at all.

I was long removed by then, but I was there the night before when husband number three died, he requested to see all of us kids, I don't know why he treated me horrible, I was sent away under his hand, for threatening to tell the truth of my mother's part in her husband's death, the man wasn't too smart, he should have been listening with his ears and not his penis in the fall of 1976, when he desired to quickly marry his dead cousin's wife. Because I did return on request and I could see his end was not so glorious either, and the lies he helped mother tell about grandma and grandpa so I couldn't go back, where I could be celebrated and loved when mother gave me a way to the state of Nebraska with no place to go, (I learned years later that he knew the system for getting rid of unwanted kids because he had done this to his own daughter a few years before to get out of paying child support.) Karma has a way of solving things, there is nothing to feel or do, just wait, it will all resolve itself.

I didn't care what he wanted, but I must admit I was curious, he was about to meet God and he was guilty, he was clearing his own conscious, after seeing that man I walked out on the front porch and said to one of my sisters, he will be dead tomorrow, he was, and by the time we arrived everything he owned was burning in a pile in the back yard, including the bed he died on.

We kids predicted the deaths before they happened, and we knew we couldn't prove it. So, we just didn't do anything, but rumor has it the last life insurance company didn't pay, premiums were received back and that was it. Like I said it was a rumor, either way, it simply didn't matter. I was no longer watching.

I wasn't sorry that Stepfather #1 died, I didn't sit with the family that day at the funeral, we were a family divided all over the place, one sister ran out and left, and after returning to the house she told me that the day they found him hanging, mom told her to stay inside, there was something bad outside, how did mom know that?

How did she know that she needed to stay inside and something bad was out in our playhouse?

She had just gotten home, and it happened while she was away, so how did she know? My sister followed my mother out the door anyway and saw our stepfather hanging there by the neck in our playhouse with his belt around his neck, just hanging there, I tell you this as I remember her telling me so many years ago, I wasn't sad because he was a mean Son of a Bitch, the only time he was nice to me was one time when he was divorced from my mother that few months, but he married her again and part of the deal I guess was to treat me like a red-headed stepchild.

I was sad for his 6-year-old, my little sister who he loved and doted on, but I was free of his knuckle wraps on my head, him looking at me in the bathroom, making fun of me because I didn't have a period yet, for me it was good residence I thought.

He didn't seem to notice his other 2-year-old, but I did, and I loved her very much until she took her own life, even though I only saw her at grandma's occasionally over the years.

However, little did I know he was harmless compared to Mother's next pick of men, what was coming was the ultimate crazy, little did mother know how guilty it made her look.

But as I stated before husband # 3 ended up dead also. So did husband #4 but I think he died of something normal, I only saw him once, he was crabby and controllable just the kind of stud my mama loved.

When he died, I didn't bother to attend, I had quit going to the funerals of my mother's dead husbands by then, a family member told me I needed to attend because it made it look as if something was wrong within the family. I said something "is" wrong and stayed home.

I no longer wanted to be associated with them, I didn't want to sit and be angry at all the names that were forged to the desired father of my mother's children, the lies on paper were public record, but they were still lies, a stranger none the wiser, but for those of us who knew, it was embarrassing, and I had learned to turn a blind eye to my mother's rewriting of history so she could claim the next batch of people that suited her as my relatives.

Grandma used to say you can fool some of the people some of the time, but no one fools everyone, every time.

One of the #1 stepfathers' cousins wrote dear old mom a letter and said he loved her, they met once at a funeral, years earlier, they just knew they were in love with one another then but couldn't do anything about it, right I thought, and yes! of course, she would marry him!

He became husband #3, Crazy right? She didn't even know him! They married less than three months after the mysterious death of husband #2, and less than a week after she met him again in person, then snuck out of town, didn't tell our grandparents, we were just gone. Packed up and taken to another state, taken away from everything known or perceived safe, horrified of the future. All pets are left behind.

Years later I learned through having the courage to ask questions that being a sophomore at a new school with no real crime (telling your mother you are going to tell on her is not a crime under the law, not speaking to your mother is not a crime, it could be considered disrespectful, but that is more of an opinion, but not harmful and lying for your mother under a threat leaves you simply NOT GUILTY.).

The day I was picked up from school in the fall of 1976 the Dawson County Sheriff told, me he didn't know what to do with me.

I might have to stay at the jail that night, but he would leave the door open as there was no reason in the world to lock me in, I had done nothing wrong; (yelling at your mom is not a crime, not speaking to your mom is not a crime, he told me.)

I had never been in trouble; he had never experienced anything like my mother trying to make me out to be a fruit loop and trying to make me out as a bad child.

My mother believed that if she could discredit my emotional credibility, it wouldn't matter what I told anyone because no one would believe me, however, the Dawson County Sherriff's office and County attorney did not find her credible, but they knew they needed to protect me from her, they just weren't sure why exactly.

The Sheriff said he knew by talking to me that her story wasn't true, he had called my school in Missouri, and I had not been a problem there ever. He was shocked, and I knew I couldn't tell the truth, if I did, I might never see my sisters again.

Mother lied about her parents so I couldn't go back there, at least not until they could be investigated, she did not want me around anyone I trusted, keeping me scared and anxious was in her favor, because she would be at risk and she knew it, and besides she was proving what she could do to me if I didn't cooperate.

Later in life grandma said, my mother would be the last person on earth she would want as a caretaker. She meant it. I knew she knew.

I told grandma the whole story, what happened in every word. She told me it didn't have a thing to do with me, but as long it was a secret it did. Grandma was embarrassed by her daughter's choices, I couldn't tell my story and hurt her more, I finally realized I just needed to tell it. It's really not a reflection on anyone anymore, just an awful experience that I have overcome.

One part of me was sad grandma didn't jump in and save us the other grown-up part of me understood my mother was her daughter, if something was wrong with her daughter, she couldn't say anything to protect us just the same.

She did the best she could, she didn't really have as many choices. She chose to stay out of harm's way and keep us kids out anytime she could.

Side note, my mother is still living, and she still doesn't want to see or talk to me, I am still being shunned by my immediate family for the most part. I have only seen her at family funerals. I walked by her at a family reunion once, but she left soon after I arrived, but since I was fifteen years old in 1976 nothing has changed except the people she is controlling. Children love their parents, even bad parents, I did or thought I did for a long time, it was really guilt that served no purpose, I have compassion for her but no real love, you have to truly feel love to have love, I didn't feel that I felt guilt, shame, hurt, fear, all negative things, and there is no light in negative energy.

Love lives in the light and is always celebrated. What I thought I felt was never love, now that I know what true love is, I know my maternal relationship had none of that.

I forgave her years ago and I give her grace and it is a blessing to know that nothing is expected of me in her old age. But I still choose to send prayers of love and forgive, I do it for myself.

For this, I am grateful. My other siblings don't see me because they might offend the matriarch in doing so. I was hurt for a long time about it. She always treated them much differently than she treated me, I am sure their memories are kinder than mine because I remember being hurt when I saw her kindness toward them, and I always wondered why she didn't love me that way.

Today I know your family is who you adopt, that cares about you and loves you, we pass through our parents so life can continue to support itself, our children pass through us the same way, our parents don't own us, we don't own our children, they only pass through us, my mother is unlike any of her family, who were and those living are, loving, generous, amazing, smart, educated, upstanding people.

She is the one-off, that was bound and determined to not belong to any system, and she took her children as hostages with her.

My Mother chooses differently, I made a conscious decision in a defining moment to never allow who she is to reflect on who I am and all or who I could choose to become,

Her crimes and abusive outbursts throughout my childhood are no longer a tie between my identity and who I am, I have cut the tie of grief and regret that bound me, I know here now today, that I can't make anyone more than they choose to be.

I choose not to blame others but to change my own life where I can, I know that sometimes we are not aware, but when we do know, we know to do better. It's a choice.

My three other sisters are all grown up now and they must live with their decisions just like the rest of us. I will always love them; they may be victims too.

QUESTIONS TO ASK YOURSELF & JOURNAL ABOUT:

Did a parent ever threaten you?

Were you betrayed by an adult or parent? How did they betray you?

Has a friend betrayed you?

Was the threat something life changing? How did you confront the threat?

Did you ever confront the threat? How did you forgive the action?

Is there something you have been waiting for your whole life? What is it?

Can you really expect this from this person?

CHAPTER 12

Forever Different the New Awareness

Every great dream begins with a dreamer. Always remember you have within you the strength, the patience, and the passion to reach for the stars to change the world. -Harriet Tubman

No, matter how hard I tried to not act like my parents, and no matter how hard I tried to change I seemed stuck, I was living a life that I didn't want but it was as if the harder I tried to break away, the more stuck I became. What I fought against I got more of.

Generational stickiness is what I call it. Fear to dream of where your family had never been.

I was a victim of Predictive Parenting as I read Shad Helmstetter's book about predictive parenting I knew my parents were clueless!

It was what I was living, but I didn't know it then, we become what we are told we are as small children, we don't even know we believe it, the subconscious mind, as well as the body, holds on to memory, even when the consciousness of the moment doesn't know it. It is true that if we are referred to as a nuisance, in the way, a bother, fat, a slob, or ugly, it sticks in a child's subconscious mind. It is there and we don't even know it. Until we recognize it, we can't change it.

I had to rethink everything I was ever told by my parents and decide if there was or wasn't the truth for me in those stories, if there was, what did I need to change?

More importantly, what did I want to change? Predict goodness for all the people in your life, hold everyone in high esteem, don't play God, don't judge, and keep a vibration of a healthy spirit constant, that's how you rise above the low intentions and never assume that your words won't get stuck in someone else's heart-mind, or subconscious.

I learned how I could overcome negative influences, rewrite old messages, and bombard my mind with a positive reading, it was helpful, but I was still filling my head with other people's information and not finding out much about my values and what I wanted. I did figure out that to get to me, I would need to go through me, to reveal the truth of who I am to myself, and there isn't an easier softer way to accomplish this.

I knew I had to change the files in my mind, to overcome and not give my parents and other critics who lived in my head power in my life at all.

Cleaning out the mental closets, with old inhumane rules, the cabinets with all the should' I had been programmed to feel guilty about that served everyone except myself and my own personal needs, and joyfully deleting and emptying the un-useful information.

If your soul knows it needs growth. You will seek growth and have a wanting you don't even understand until you do. I allowed my soul to be led by my highest intention, the opportunity for change. I came from a personal childhood that was a mess and was a super achiever in my career and adult life.

There was so much negativity in my mind and heart from the past that I could not make my actions align to achieve my dreams. I had to do some clearing work, I had to let go of what no longer served me. I was a super achiever at work and a super binge eater at night when I went home, sound familiar?

It was just random stuff in there, it was like cleaning out the garage, we keep certain stuff that is unusual, but we keep it, now when it comes up, I say what do I need to know here?

I would quit again every single day, but I always set myself up. I was always keeping goodies in the house for the kids, that was a justification for buying but not the truth, I was always setting up my next binge, but I didn't understand why.

If it's useful, I keep it if not I say delete it, and I had to take the responsibility to change whatever it was even if it did feel like I was being disloyal to my family. Huge subconscious triggers, living a happy life without their chaos left me feeling guilty, once I was aware of it I could defuse the trigger, not until.

Why did I care about that? Because I am not them and I do care. I watched from a distance, and I saw how karma has taken care of the historical actions, I didn't have to do anything, the law of attraction is always in play too good for good and bad for bad, and I am not able to change that law, I am grateful I understand the law. For every action, there is a reaction.

One of the craziest things I have ever thought about because my family was never loyal to me. But deep down I was loyal to them.

But it didn't matter, I choose to live in the frequency of love, kindness, joy, and generosity.

Ironically, I wanted them to still love me, (which never happened) as the years passed, when I went back, I went home to grandma and grandpa, they were the safe haven, when they were gone there was no one else to go to, except Aunt Mary, who remains my north star still to this day.

I knew I had to choose to live my own life and be okay with my choices, my family decided I was offending them in doing so, after all, each of us must live first for ourselves, we must put on our own air mask first before we can help someone else. I want for my family everything I want for myself, but I cannot do that for them, they must do their own path in this life I must do mine.

Besides, I was grown up and I wanted a different and better life for my own children, and I wasn't doing very well because my past was now stepping on my children's future. So, as I grew in awareness, I wanted everything to change for my sake and for my children, I think all parents make mistakes and some of them carry on for generations, I didn't understand my mother's choices because I knew her parents, I lived in their household at times and never received an unnecessary unkindness, sometimes I received redirection, but nothing like what I had experienced at home.

My mother complained of having to wear ugly clothes as a child, but that's not something that turns you into a monster toward your children seemingly and mostly to spite your own mother.

So instead of brown conservative clothes, she dressed us like little hookers. I didn't like to be physically exposed while wearing my mother's taste in clothes, I felt uncomfortable, she was telling me I was fat, and even though I realize now I really wasn't, I still was not ready to reveal my body to the world in hot pants and miniskirts, and oddly enough she could not hear me.

She was her mother, opposite and the same in this department. My modesty was not respected, and I still cringe when I see pictures of the flower power dresses, and the white mini dresses we were confirmed in, she was making a statement with those clothes, and I was being molested by being forced to wear them. Grandma didn't let her flaunt it, so she made me.

I asked all the simple questions like was my mother beaten, sexually abused, or mentally ill, but all were denied, and nothing was diagnosed.

My grandmother did tell me though that she had made a complaint against one of her brothers, and grandma regretted not believing her because she ran away shortly after, there were rumors that I had a brother born in Sheridan Wyoming, 1957-58 he would be in his sixty's now if there is any truth in the story, I searched old reformatory records from that event and nothing was ever found, I do know however whenever that particular uncle came around my mother did not leave us alone with him, he had usually been drinking, and he never got past the front porch, that I remember. I never knew if she protected us from the overly Huggy drunk or something else. I am glad she chose to protect us.

Children live the results found in the files of their subconscious minds, even if you are not aware the programming is there, I know it was true for me.

The files were the ingrained habits and rules, and I lived what was safe to me even though it was chaotic, it was all I knew.

My files were given to me by someone else, mostly useless information, and everything that was holding me back was the first 16+ years of programming. I was born with an empty closet and now my closet was full of mostly the wrong files. Other people's conditioning and opinions are not mine for my life.

Every decision I had ever made up to that point was based on those files stored in my subconscious mind. My life outcome to date was a result of those files. Everything I believed about myself, up to this point is a result of those stored files. Every conscious change I have aligned to love, and kindness has changed my choices, what was available to me, and how I felt about everything. The physical illness left, and health returned with each act of consciousness, where the mind goes the body follows.

My parent's negative, abusive, and neglective lifestyle and treatment were my guidance system for a computer-like program that set my attitude, speed, and direction, to the worst possible destination. Every binge-eating episode left me with low to no self-worth. Every starvation week left me reeling for joy, but it couldn't last, I knew that the alcoholic could put the cap on the bottle, but I had to let the tiger out of the cage and eat every day to live.

I had received very bad directions! When I asked questions about why or resisted or tried to tell them how I felt they threw their God at me and talked forgiveness and harmony. Nothing controlling and suppressive of the soul can set it free to become what the creator intended it to be. I tried to white-knuckle it and fight it all the way, but the harder I fought the more I got. My eating and binges diminished in my surrender that I couldn't control it, something, or someone else could, I must let them.

Yet I surrendered and it worked. I didn't know how or why but that decision cleared the path for the clarity that followed.

Man's doctrines about the creator's rules are just about control, taught from generation to generation, mostly because that's the way it was always done.

Neither of my parents ever said they were sorry or that they were wrong, I am sure they never will, and the forgiveness I offer is my own freedom, silently and quietly. I hold nothing against them because I do believe they were working with what they personally knew in my raising. They are forgiven and free of any obligation to me, they may have had to deal with themselves at some point, but I am not aware. I just want them to feel good and enjoy life now. True wellness comes when you can want for others what you want for yourself.

I forgive people who apologize sincerely, I don't walk around forgiving people who don't, however, I don't hold a grudge either, I just let that go, as unimportant, and even when people do apologize to me that does not mean that I trust them, that's an earned state of privilege, and I have seen nothing in my lifetime that tells me to trust my mother, and I have a very guarded trust with my father. I love my dad, but I really don't trust him fully, mostly because my dog doesn't, and I trust my dog's instincts more than my own.

For a long time, I believed I was what my parents told me I was, I lived the life they carved out for me in their expectations or lack of expectations for sure, what I know here now today is that human experience is a state of mind. I look back at the illusiveness of it all, it's real but has no power, just experiences of old memories.

The largest illusion of humankind we do not recognize and realize that we are made in God's highest form of creation, I did not realize I am made in the highest image of God, I had to realize that all the causes of our life are due to my own state of consciousness. What I remembered and how I remembered, others can be at the same event and remember it differently, there is no one to discredit about this, each person has their own memory and their own truth. This story is my memory.

When I no longer told my parent's version of my life's stories to myself my life changed.

I don't tell you this to blame or shame anyone, I tell you now so you can know how it was for me, what happened and how it is now. Maybe your story is similar, we all need to know we are not alone, others have suffered, others have overcome food additions and binge eating, no one else can tell us what we are, we must each decide for ourselves and start our own recovery accordingly.

If you choose to live in a negative story, you have a negative attitude and life, when we change our attitude to a positive, loving, and giving attitude you are able to receive positive and good things. I am living proof of this.

I know you are probably wondering, does she even believe in God, of course, I do, I believe in the one that existed before anyone tried to market it or make living preaching about it, altering it. The Alpha and the Omega, the beginning, and the end.

There is only one, we each have our own path to get to God, I believe the infinite creator is the light that lives in each one of us, each path is acceptable to this great entity of infinite grace love, and power, the moment you say yes in love, kindness, and joy you are there, it lives in you, it's your spirit always with you, take good care of it.

My lack of self-esteem left me feeling unworthy of anything good since my self-esteem was practically nonexistent, everything I believed about myself was based on those old files, and someone else's lies, how I was treated, how I was thrown away, how I was offered up as meat to men by my mother as a child by age 12, her first offering was one of her own high school boyfriends, I was mortified she wanted me to talk sexy to him on the phone when she handed me the phone I was speechless, I wanted to please my mother, but I did not want this grown man to be my boyfriend!

I have the courage to say today what I prefer in all situations; I ask for what I want. I know I can have what I desire. Whether it be something as simple as food, or as important as where I live and the house, I live in.

I told grandma what had happened, the planned parenthood saga and the boyfriends, only to get in trouble once again for the blabbing of the family business, but grandma must have told her how I felt because my mother didn't ever want to talk to me for a long time, her silence was one of her punishments, she often had men in the house waiting to meet us girls when we arrived home from school, and they were men of the worst kind, why did she want to make sure we lost our virginity? Why was that so important to her? I guess I will never know. But its sick.

I never regretted telling, I gave myself a chance every time I found my voice and did what I believed was right.

Why was this peculiar control so important to her?

I know that I will never know what her influence was, but I do know that I have no regrets, and today I realize how much I did love myself by speaking out. I realize how grateful I am that I was a courageous and tenacious child. It made me a bold beautiful courageous woman.

How could she sacrifice her little girls to the white trash trailer scum? I will never know that answer.

My own value was about how I felt every time one of my siblings died in a tragic accident, when other kids were home safe with their families, by the time my fourth sibling had died needlessly my mind was so overwhelmed, I felt survivor guilt for escaping.

How I felt after the suicide of my sister that I could not find the day she died when no one would help me find her, I called everyone, but no one had time, their baby was asleep, but I will bet if they needed to go pick up their husband from work they would have woke up that baby, she said she would look for her after her baby woke up, she didn't.

The lack of care about this sister was stifling my emotional ability to cope, she and I had become very close in her few years in Nebraska, and I knew her well enough to know that something was seriously wrong.

My sister who was too busy to do this small errand of life or death later said you might have an issue with me because I didn't go look for her after the baby woke up, no I didn't have an issue, I was 10 hours away, she was 30 minutes by the time I figured it out, she has to take responsibility for her choices now, I had done all I could do, I did do all I could, none the less she walked into a train 3 hours later, from a quarter of a mile away, there was no stopping that loaded freight train, she walked near as possible, waved goodbye to the engineer, turned her back to that train died 14 minutes later, I empathetically felt the physical pain of her death with those details, in her suicide note where she said: "if heaven is so wonderful why would I want to stay here?"

With the response of my family, and how she was only 22, beautiful, and feeling unloved and unwanted, there is no way I did not understand her suicide note statements, I didn't agree with them, but I had lived them, and I understood. She escaped I remained trapped.

She had her picture taken for me to pick up at Walmart, something to make sure we remembered her, I did, and still do.

The following year I gained over 100 pounds as I choked down the emotions that went with the reality that my family would never care for anyone other than themselves. When my mother said I didn't expect her to do anything else, but never ever tried to help her, just justified that it was always going to happen as though it ran in the family I wanted to puke, I remembered all over again the day her father died the day I lied. And my mother continues to weave justification into the acts of her daughter to justify the suicide she stories she fed my sister since the supposed suicide of her father in our playhouse, you know it runs in families, it's just the way it is malarky. For every action, there is always, always, always, a reaction.

People do things because other people made it acceptable. Tell me I am fat long enough and I will believe you and become fat. Oh, that already happened.

Beliefs separate people, but values bring them together, my family didn't value one another, they destroyed each other, and they enjoyed it like Saturday night wrestling.

It all had to do with what I did, said, and how I acted because until I could undo and overcome what had been done to me, by others, by myself, and by the ridiculous rules, I didn't have a chance.

It all started to change when I realized I could make conscious choices and take responsibility for my own life so that I could change my reality, so that is what I started doing. I looked for progress, not perfection, but every day I took care of myself a little bit better than the day before.

Unfortunately, I wasn't a perfect mother and by now my own kids were in their late teens and no longer lived at home.

I was doing everything I could to do the right thing for them, but it wasn't all perfect, and still isn't, but maybe perfect is an egotistical myth.

I've learned that it's not how we judge that matters, it's that we judge, it is not how we blame that matters, it's that we blame, it's not how we justify, but that we justify, it's not how we were shamed, it's that we continue to shame, it's not how others see us, it's how we see ourselves, it is not how we see ourselves, it's how we are seen by our creator, to be in opposition is to be in battle with the creator, the creator is a part of me and I am a part of it. I no longer fight myself. I love and accept myself.

Today I chose to live within the gift of imperfection, I tried being what everyone else wanted, doing what everyone else wanted, I lived the suggestions of others, and they didn't notice, and I was miserable, I want to be a bit of a bad girl sometimes, vicarious pleasure has a place in my life. It's called living.

There are no rituals that are right or wrong. Every person has the right to choose their own way if they are not hurting anyone else in doing so. Love is not a criminal act unless you are a stalker!

And even in that no one needs to tell us if it comes up, we each have our own innate sense of right and wrong, in our own heart if something is wrong or hurtful, I just choose the opposite, if it comes up in your heart as okay, it is, what bothers one person may not bother another today, later it may or not.

It is not how we express our anger, it's that we need to express it at all. Sometimes we need to use our words, I just choose to not say anything until I can say it as diplomatic and kindly as possible, not 100% but better than it used to be.

I am grateful we all have different DNA, if something doesn't sit right with you about someone else it is not your job to change them, it's not your job to judge how you think they should, be, think or do, however either. In fact, we are all perfect just the way we are.

And no, you don't have to say anything to them, and you can be in the same room with them, quietly observe and sit where you want.

Most people want to love, be loved, and have peace. If they don't, they are not where I am anyway. Because I am free to go anytime, I choose today.

Ever since that realization I have been reprogramming my files. Re- examining the old stories, cleaning out the old file cabinets, throwing out negative messages, and replacing them with positive outcomes and kindness to myself, and as a result to others.

I moved on and made positive changes, other people in my life and family are still stuck on that old never changing hamster wheel, it's okay, I don't need to play on that cage or spend time with people who bring down my vibration, in fact, I keep my vibration so high that when those storms come through these days I hardly notice. I do notice that makes those wave makers very angry sometimes, but that's their business, not mine.

You can't give what you don't have, I try to live in appreciative gratitude and joy every single today.

I meditate, I hear God's voice through my own intuition, and send love to those who sometimes bother me emotionally. I receive all good blessings that come to me, I am worthy, I am loved, and I am not alone even without my family, I AM here, I AM living gratefully, and I AM loved.

I have replaced traditional activities with adventures, some of the traditional things in my life were emotional events like family holidays and reunions, I have my own tribe, and I accept that life passes through us and moves on around us.

As a parent I felt like I failed my children in many ways because I was listening to the opinion of others on how they should be raised, I was not listening to my inner voice and trusting my own intuition, and I didn't learn much of this till my children were 9+ years old, my life wasn't good.

But I know with all my heart I did the best I could, and when I did start to know better, I began to do better, but even children resist change, their ego is not much different than the adult ego. Just faster physically.

I married the first two men who gave me any attention at all because I didn't believe I could do any better, my children had different fathers, and I chose not to marry either of them. I have no regrets, I only regretted the two unnecessary marriages, that I was shamed into, I would have been perfectly fine as a single woman raising my children, there are no bastards in the world. A name is not something you are it's something you have.

There was nothing to be ashamed of about that, if someone throws shame at another person it is theirs, not the person they are throwing it at.

What others told me was their belief and reality, not mine, it was mine when I believed them, it is my life, and it is not anyone else's business, their good intentions were not good intentions!

My morality was fine, and their bible has a hell of a lot of sex, concubines, murder, and wars because people wouldn't believe as the king desired not to mention polygamy in it! More people have been killed over religion than from natural disasters.

Let us call it being human, simple experiences that eventually help us get to the life and personal values we are intended to live. It is neither right nor wrong, just real-life stuff.

We are not separate from the divine force or from one another, we are not separate, and our realization of unity comes at a cost of the decision to grow and become separate we are not really forced to choose that is something we do. An action we take. When we choose separation, we put ourselves in isolation.

Today I have no regrets about my own choices, only following the directions and expectations of others who sought to control me and my children. It was not how I needed approval; it was that I needed approval.

My insecurity put people who were not good fits or mates, and often they weren't even good lovers into my life! Today I would look you over and think to myself do I really want you to crawl around on me? Slobber on me, sweat on me, all of this in my life, if only I was taught to stand up for myself and do what I thought was best for myself, my body, my being, and allowed to believe that it was okay to think for myself, all these lacks stopped my own identity and trickled unfortunately to my children, an unintended multigenerational experience. It was not how or with whom we have sex; it is that we thought it was needed to be whole.

I didn't need to do anything against myself at my parent's suggestion as an adult I was simply conditioned to it, as children we often have no choices, I do now.

My children do now, I have done my best to lead by example, allowing them to take what has value to them and spit out the bones, it's the best I can do. It is not how we decide to be perfect; it is what we think we need to be.

All the limiting beliefs that told me I was not good enough, I was wrong, I was stupid, I was ignorant, and I could not make good decisions for myself, if I found my voice, and opened my mind, I would tell the truth of how it was, I am.

It was not that I thought I wasn't enough; it was that I AM known and give permission of awareness to the truth. I AM a piece of source; the Source is a piece of me. I call Source God.

It's a relief to tell my truth. My perception may be different than others who were there at the time of my experiences and that's okay, we all hear things and experience them differently, and that's their truth. And I chose to not be offended.

I accept that others get to keep their memories and thoughts in the comfortable space they prefer, the discomfort of my soul brought me here, I do not inject it into my life as somehow doing so would change theirs. It wouldn't, I can only change my life and look at my own perceptions. Everyone else must do that part for themselves also. It is not that we have memories; it is that we do with the knowledge of this illusion. The memory fades and softens with love and caring.

My Other Grandma Echo, the one I was named after died when I was 13, I was heartbroken, I loved dressing up and having tea parties on her front porch. I knew she was sick, but I didn't think she was going to die. All my memories of her were good, we ate pickles and cookies at her house, walked to the store to see Swag and bought ice cream, and slept slumber party style together.

My feelings were stuck inside me, I couldn't say anything, they took me to the funeral home again to see the dead body but not to the funeral, so I really didn't hear the message of what happened when you transcend and leave this earth, you were just dead. It is not that I am dead; it is that understanding that I have transcended into a higher vibration, and I do not need to be sad; it was that I believed sadness and grief were required.

I remember wanting to look at her closer, other people touched her, I was afraid to do anything, that big old two-story funeral home seemed to have a lot of rooms. Everyone was standing around talking and telling stories, I am not sure where my mother was, I might have gone with grandma because I don't remember any drama, just quiet, and lots of families that acted like family to one another.

I was raped at 14 years of age, I never told a soul, I was petrified it would happen again, years later when I had the abdominoplasty, the procedure removed 17 pounds of skin from my lap but also left my surgeon quite disturbed. I decided to be a donor to the burn center with that skin and help others not have to suffer skin grafting in the burn unit at the hospital a few days after the procedure the surgeon came in to talk to me with some very uncomfortable questions. It was not that there was a past; it was a past trapped in my body. My body may have been overtaken physically but I refuse to give a rapist or an abuser my mind also. That person is not well enough equipped to have a battle of wits with me. I will win every time.

He said he had never seen anything like this before, when he put my skin on the donor board to go to the donor center there was a perfect bite mark, human, and very severe scar tissue around it, it disturbed him, but it disturbed me too. When I was 14, I was raped and my attacker bit me on the stomach and told me if I ever told anyone he would kill me. I don't know why I didn't tell other than I was scared. It was not how I was afraid; it was that I believed fear had a right to place itself and dwell in me.

He told his stepbrother and other boys, and they taunted me, I was bullied and afraid all the time, his brother shot me with a bee-bee gun on the way home and told me it will be worse than this if you tell, we'll all get you! It was not how I was bullied; it was that I believed I deserved it.

The next Sunday in church I broke down, I did not believe there was a God that could love me because if there was why did he let all this stuff happen to me? I hadn't missed a Sunday for years and I refused to go after that, what good was God if he didn't protect me from all the evil around me? It wasn't how I questioned God; it was that I believed he was outside myself, I am a piece of God, God is a piece of me.

I told my surgeon the story and he hung his head and said I think you are one of the strongest survivors I have ever met. Rightly so. And we never talked about it again.

When I was 15 my stepfather died, and at I was 16 and caught in the middle of a lot of lying and deception, which carried a lot of guilt and fear again, the lies and secrets around this man's death were haunting to most anyone who was or is close enough to know a little bit about truth, human nature is if we don't talk about it, we forget about it, we don't, our subconscious mind is powerful and our body keeps score, and our loss is often ourselves in these secrets and lies. It was not how the secret came to be; it was that I believed a secret necessary.

Fact-finding has been my greatest core value throughout my life because of the lies and secrets surrounding this man, I didn't even like him, but his death changed my life forever.

My mother gave me a way to the state of Nebraska before just giving your kids away was accepted or popular, and yet she did me a favor, under her tutelage I would perhaps never have sought out the answers for my life, it would have more than likely been discouraged.

Mother never liked anyone to know something that she did not know. However, she was living in a world only as big as her education and imagination, and from where I sat it didn't look like something I wanted for myself.

I was extremely young and at age 16 when I was pregnant with my first child, (not surprising with the statistics of at-risk children today with my type of past, but much rarer in the 1960s and 1970s).

Since my mother had given me away before she knew a child was involved, she had no real control, and once I was found to be pregnant the state of Nebraska Emancipated me. Hooray! Now what?

This little child I carried, I loved him and wanted the best for him, better than I could give him a chance to have a good family, enough of everything, a family to love him not just be there to feed and water him, since I was in an unwed mother's home and planned on allowing him to be adopted by good parents who would love and provide for him since my mother had thrown me away, but now my mother was trying to intervene now and adopt my baby. It was not how I controlled; it was that I needed to.

I had no place to go after my baby was born, except back under my mother's roof, she did not want me there, so she bought a little house for me and the baby to stay in it. That house paved the way to many disasters, and many joys.

One door in and one door out. I was terrified of being alone at night, and of course, I had no income, but my mother could get social security on me through her dead murdered husband, she gave me $150 each month, but it would run out at 18 years of age, so I had better be getting a man to support me. It was not how I was supported; it was that I believed that I should be supported by others' ideas. It was not how I was married; it was only the thought that it was needed. It was not a reason to ruin so many lives.

Why wasn't she helping me get an education and a good job, oh, it wasn't part of her blueprint for my life, if I wanted anything that elaborate, I would have to figure it out for myself.

I cannot tell you how that enraged me, she got a new husband and because I said out loud, I did not like him, and I was going to tell the entire story of how her and junkyard boyfriend killed her last husband, she gave me away. It was not how I found my voice; it was that it was needed.

And now she was going to adopt my baby, over my dead body I thought, in those days in the family adoption happened a lot, so to stop her I ended up going home with a child that I was in no way equipped to care for. I just knew in her hands he would not survive, so many of us didn't.

I loved him, and still do he is 45 years old this year, and he shines like the son he is, but could I have loved him better by letting strangers raise him, I don't know, I didn't find that out, I chickened out and took the life sentence I was given in the circumstance that was served up, but he loves me, and I love him, and that's all that really matters, and I believe I did better than my parents, however, I did not know what I didn't know.

When my first child was seven months old when I became pregnant the second, I was seventeen, I didn't know what to do and her father was more than willing to pay for an abortion, I went to the appointment, but never went in, and I couldn't do it. I didn't know what I was going to do, so 3 weeks later I married a man that worked at the mill with my mother's new husband, great my mother picked him out, I didn't have a choice I felt, my back was against the wall, and I didn't know if I could keep my baby, so I married a man who drank, smoked and ran around more than 10 years older than me. It was not how it happened; only that I believed it needed to happen at all.

It was not a happy union, it was miserable, it was not uncommon that he gambled away his paycheck before the bank opened on payday, we moved every couple of months because we couldn't pay the bills due to the drinking and gambling, I was trapped in a cage without bars, and I wanted out! It wasn't what happened it was my perception. For a moment in life I believed I didn't have a choice.

To make life super interesting I had no money, no place to go, no one to trust, and it was perceived to be the trouble of my own making, so since that was the attitude of my parents, I took full responsibility for the next time he came home drunk and broke.

I gave him a fifth of whiskey, waited for him to pass out, loaded everything in the house, and left, and yes, I left him without clothes, without anything. I felt better.

That same summer was the first time I started really being a parent and understanding how to parent and nurture my own children they were 2 and 3 now, and how to be a mom, and there weren't lessons for people who were not abusing their kids, but grandma helped me.

I started talking to my kids with real conversations, my mom never talked to me, she talked toward me, I started reading to my kids, providing regular meals instead of feeding when they were hungry like when they were still bottle feeding, and their behaviors were because of what I didn't know and have myself, and they threw fits, we're not potty training well, and I realized they needed my attention just like I need my mother's only differently, and I did not know how to not be manipulated, I had to learn what was manipulation before I could defend against it, I had to learn what was considered normal and what was not, then I could recognize it and say no, and the acting out stopped.

I had no idea what a normal relationship was, and still don't, but I think if love, joy, and respect are included it is probably normal enough.

Husband #1 and I were separated 17 times over 5 years and the last time I left his clothes on his mother's roof, while he lay naked in a trailer house 11 miles away without a way to call or get to anything he needed, that would have been something my mother would have done I felt ashamed at the time, but looking back I am glad I finally did something, anything to change my life, start a new direction.

All I knew was his carousing around was over, I was done. I could not live in an open marriage which was what he preferred. He and my mother would have gotten along great.

Husband # 2 was so nice until 15 minutes after our wedding and then he went into ownership mode.

What a prick, my ex-husband had adopted my first child and claimed my second as we were married when she was born, and he and I actually parted friends, husband #2 was extremely jealous and could not stand that I decided to be an adult and be sociable with my x-husband and because we were friends, he wanted to adopt my kids and cut my ex-husband out of the picture, I didn't like the idea my kids had their identity and I wanted to leave things the way they were.

He wouldn't leave it alone, he acted as though he was going to be the best dad in the world, and my first husband was paying support for 2 kids that weren't his, and I felt guilty about that, the shame of my past was working well then, but today I would never allow it, but it is because of the pain and learning for myself and my children and what we went through because of my need for his approval, but I did want to give him relief financially today I would just write the check back to him each month, and let him love those kids and those kids love him because finally, I allowed my kids to be adopted and 20 minutes later he proved to be the worst dad in the world.

But I did let him go to jail for being the worst dad in the world. And I would do it again. I am not a needy co-dependent woman today (by then I obviously wasn't either). It doesn't hurt to call it what it is and remove yourself from all people who are of a harmful mindset, no matter who they are.

Why did I think we would be one big happy family? It was just a dream I guess, no, an illusion, he was horrible to "his" children as he saw fit now that he had his papers, I wanted out and still had no way to support my kids, I had worked off and on, but the son of a bitch could not make a sandwich and stuff it in his head himself, so I decided to go to beauty school and become a cosmetologist, he said what I am I going to do for lunch, I said put a piece of meat between 2 pieces of bread and stick it in your head or starve to death, I really don't care. It is not how you escape; it is the need to escape.

Grandma gave me a thousand dollars for graduating from beauty school and there was a salon for sale under bankruptcy, I bought that business for $500 and furnished the inventory with the rest, it is still paying me today, I built assets, friendships, colleagues, and alliances with that money and with the next abusive situation, I divorced that him while he was in jail.

By now all I wanted was out, it was years later that I discovered that he had been stalking me. And I was clueless, I wasn't looking for that kind of behavior in my own naivety and so I didn't even notice him. I should have but I didn't.

My second ex-husband did everything he could to come between me and my children, and they learned how to come between us, there was no punishment for him until jail and I would not settle for anything less, but if he would have died, I would have looked at the world as a better place.

He was horrible for my children and for me, my pride would never allow me to go to a welfare system for any reason, now I wish I would have, at least my kids would have been safe, intact and we could have always remained together. I know that every abuser separates and divides first, I saw it as a child, but I did not recognize it. It was not how I flew away; only that I discovered I could.

My daughter, unfortunately, had to sit out the back burner a lot of times while meeting the needs of her brother, who my ex-husband was working to destroy over time, who already had his own issues with his disability, my daughter is more me than I am myself, so if your reading this thinking I have a gutsy punch, she is one up on me, this is one thing which has made us closer at times and far apart at times, but it's part of life's cycle I think, and I think she knows I am never very far away, we must let our children be themselves and try not to hurry them into adulthood, if I could do anything differently I would not have allowed her to get married young, I was worried she would choose to get a pregnant as a way of escaping, so I gave in and let her get married at 16, I cannot say that would have been a solution to a problem today, they were married 6 years before the first daughter was born, I was glad she was not a baby having babies. It is not how history is changed; just that there is a new way.

She had 4 children and a twenty-year marriage before it ended. Those old generational beliefs were still guiding me then, now I know that it would not have mattered, but she was honorable and did get her high school education as a married woman, with honor.

She knew how to follow through and I am grateful that she did. She proved to be a survivor like me, I only wish that while I was looking for a way out of our life, it would not have left her a victim of the life I was trying so hard to escape.

Then she was finally mad at her mom about everything, and that was okay too. She was in her cycle of growth as a woman, and I knew it, I know we do not grow in comfort but in adversity.

We don't welcome it, but usually, it looks different when we look back on it. I love my children, and I have no regrets about the freedom I gave up, I did choose to have a tubal ligation procedure at age 19 after my daughter was born because I knew I did not want more children, I wanted to be able to care for the two I had efficiently, financially, and I was an uneducated young woman with two small children, my now ex-husband and I were separated at the time, and we had medical insurance, grandma paid the $500 deductible and I chose to have this permanent procedure done, I never wanted to have another baby, my mother heard about it and told everyone I had an abortion, no I didn't but if I was pregnant again I might have chosen too, and it would have been my choice, I did it. because I wanted to make sure I didn't, have any more children ever. I had no regrets; no shame, it was my first attempt at owning my own body.

Free at last, free at last, I took my half of the sale of my house and me and my daughter got an apartment nearby, my son was 18 and off running the world by then, or so he would tell you, I remember the first night in that little apartment, having supper there, she and I both stuck our fork in the butter at the same time, we had come out on the other side. All the bullshit controlling rules were done and over with!

I left a convenient financial situation to protect my children, the sad thing is I truly loved him once, and he betrayed me in so many ways with unimaginable things, but once I knew the truth, I was not about to make excuses for him, I was out of there, I wanted my children to have peace and be okay.

It was a long road, but today everyone is safe under their own roof, and I know I did the best I could and started over one more time. Hindsight is always 20/20, our lives are not mistakes, they are a series of experiences and some of them we do to ourselves, some of it is done to us and beyond our control, and some of us are just trying to move past whatever is in the way of our heart, one thing I know is the heart wants, what the heart wants.

And when this is true, and bound in truth, the pain of getting relief from everything that holds you back is worth it. It has been for me, and I know that I have never regretted the day I mustered up the courage and went for it. You can to. What scares you the most will be your greatest triumph.

It was my time, and I wasn't very responsible for a while, I had never been a young adult, had friends, been barhopping, going shopping for new clothes, made my own money, and had a job that wasn't getting us more than from pay check to pay check, this freedom was different to me and I loved it, I lived for it, I was finding out my personal values, learning more, seeking more, asking more of myself and nothing was unacceptable, and I wanted to do it all, my weight came down and men were coming around, I was like my mother I guess I could always attract a bad man. It was not who I attracted; only that I needed to attract.

But I was a quick learner, I would say to myself, do you want this to crawl on you at night, and I found myself saying nope, and the bar days were done.

I found other things to do, I took my kids to the petting zoo, botanical gardens, and out to eat a meal, I went away for weekends and allowed myself to enjoy life, I learned and decided with each experience if it was something I wanted to do again or not, but I tried, I could pay my own way and I was not an ignorant child or adult, I could learn and I did, and the more awareness I cultivated in my life the more blowback I received in my family, I was considered too big for my britches, unholy, unworthy, unwilling to play by the old family rules. (Never did really).

I was the one who was willing to let the truth set me free, I became willing to burn the ships and exhume the bodies. I am the master of my fate and the captain of my soul. If I made a mistake, I chose another way the next time.

I ran my business and went to lunch, joined a couple of book clubs, and found that life had so much richness to offer through literature and learning, I stood behind the chair and inspired other young cosmetologists to become champions in the industry also, and yes, I attracted the broken and unwanted. It was not how they came, only that they be raised upon arriving.

And yes they are successful today because I had the courage to lead by example and love the way I wanted to be loved, and I also smile when I drive by the salon they work at or own, because I know I was a part of them growing from a new stylist in the business, even the ones who left on poor terms always eventually reached out to make amends, my response is non-needed, I wish you all the best blessings on your life, and I appreciate you taking this time for yourself because I know and understand the value of completing the incompletes in life. It is not how we learn but knowing we can.

We cannot make the people we apologize to in life accept our apologies for our part in apology is about how we acted or reacted, we can only clear our side of the street, I learned that with my mother, what she does or doesn't do with the information is 100% her responsibility, but we can clear our own driveways, and live differently, it's sometimes hard, but whatever comes to mind for you when you think about it is what you probably need to take care of.

It is not something you should just go out and do, if you slept with a friend's husband telling her is only beneficial to you, it would hurt her, so meditate on everything, look at your personal motives and talk to someone who can help you think it all the way through. You don't need to be Catholic to see a priest but if you want the secrets of your mind and out of your conscious, I recommend one, they won't even tell God. And can tell no one anything ever.

Then if the opportunity is provided, apologize with only the best interest of the other person and no regard for yourself, but have regard for your family, the outcome, or consequences, if you owe something pay it, if you stole something redeem it with interest, be complete.

I always told my kids, before you do something think it all the way through, how will this decision affect others, and will you put yourself in a different light, if so, is the light good or negative, is this selfish? self-centered? Are reactions going to be worth it in the end? Or does this decision have value and joy for the universe and your life? It is not how we create good; it is that the good we create reaches wide in our world.

I finally cut the manipulation link with about everyone in my life, those were turbulent times when this mom got a backbone and stopped being manipulated and pushed even by her own children, that unexpected behavior. At least in my own home, what others do elsewhere is their personal business, my kids are grown up and I wasn't perfect, and they weren't either, I worry my grandchildren will be caught in the crossfire and it will go another generation, the crossfire is nothing but life, every action has a reaction, every word brings another thought, but that will be their choice, we all have a choice. I am only responsible for my behavior.

Events will always happen in our lives, we cannot control everything and especially other people, we can only choose how we do or don't react to those events, and if we think it through before we react, we will likely have more favorable outcomes as life moves forward.

And if we don't get what we would prefer doing the right thing, it does not mean we are wrong or unsuccessful, we are just dealing with people who are not ready yet, or perhaps just the wrong people, we will always find our tribe if we look long enough, hard enough, and care enough.

But if we don't find our tribe we are not alone, Divine God is a part of you and you are a part of it, and if we did the next right thing we are always way ahead of the game.

My children are grown and responsible for their children, I am sorry I did not know more to do better, but I did the best I could with what I had.

And I can honestly say I never woke up any morning of my life and did anything intentionally to hurt anyone, not my children or my family, I simply write the truth for me from my perception of what happened and my personal memory and experience.

I wish I could say the same about my parents, they came from better and did the opposite. They have their own story also, I guess it was a statement they were making. I just happened to be another kid born to young parents who they turned into their victims.

I did know that my own future was at stake, their crazy lives made my life overwhelming. And again, they were just simply unaware, or I hope they were because to believe it was all intentional against me would really be potentially painful, the world is only as big as it is in their minds, for my parents the world is only as big as their own vision and that vision seems small from where I sit. It is not how I come to see the world; it is that I find vision.

The subconscious mind will accept and store anything it is told whether it is true or not. That's the beauty of life if we want to believe a lie about ourselves or someone else we can, it is so easy to stay in our comfort zone, but it is far more difficult to accept and receive the truth, that's why often it is said that the truth hurts, but it also heals, my mother was a woman who was who she was, and I unexpectedly followed in her footsteps in some ways unintentionally, but I also have had to look at my part in my life, my choices, my incompletes, and my victories, which have been harder to receive and except because of what I believed about myself deep down, receiving the good the world had to offer for me was one of the most powerful confirmations of self-love and worthiness that I could ever do!

Telling myself good things about myself I felt like an impostor at first, when I thought about writing I first told myself I wasn't qualified, I had graduated from nothing, but I did write that first unpublished book, but because my self-esteem was so low, I did not recognize it as a victory.

Now I AM an international bestselling Amazon Author.

I went back and finished high school, but the shame of not finishing hid that victory for many, many, years. I went to cosmetology school, owned a business, and helped others succeed for almost 25 years, another victory, I raised 2 children pretty much single-handedly and they can make their own way today, another victory!

I worked as a financial advisor for the last 12 years and gifted my practice to another agent to allow him to succeed! Another victory!

After two failed marriages I met the sweetheart of my life and we will be married 25 years in July, he is a kind gentleman who loves me for me. And we adopted a puppy 2 years ago and he is a joy and bundle of unconditional love, what a joy to recognize that I have turned out to be an awesome human being!

I have taken the lemons in my life and made lemonade every time! I own it today as I should!

I remember thinking, wow, I have made so many mistakes how do I know what is right? Today I don't even believe in mistakes, I believe in experiences, and I have had some no doubt, but I learned from them and that is called living life, to not learn is to live as a fool.

When life has been extremely negative how do you think up good things to tell yourself? You read! I read everything I could put my hands on, and I started realizing I was abused by others and what abuse was, but I also realized that I was abusing myself because of the beliefs I had about myself that others had given to me through the conditions and belief systems that were likely in place for generations, we do it because some did it before no other reason other than that's the way we always did it.

Every story became a Metaphor for my own personal growth, it was a story in the past, I resolved it and if it came back up, I resolved it again.

The more I rethought the stories, especially without telling them and giving others power to judge them the more I found out how important it was to re-examine what they were.

Here and now the less power they have, that's what makes me a passionate keynote speaker, and teacher today, that's where the real breakthroughs are, that's where we find out what's holding someone back, we examine the somethings and find out what is true.

QUESTIONS TO ASK YOURSELF AND JOURNAL ABOUT:

Do you feel like you are living your own life? What did you dream of becoming as a child?

Who told you it was silly, and you could not?

What do you want now?

Pretend you do know, what would it be?

Were you conditioned by others and stuck in a life you don't want right now?

If so, what is one thing you could do to change your circumstances today?

If you did how would that change the way you feel about your life? Can You Give yourself permission to change?

Did a parent ever use a bad thing someone else did to justify their choices and actions toward you?

If so, what did they do or say that hurt you then?

In abusive neglective Homes gaslighting is often used against children, look it up, can you relate the definition to your own experiences?

How do you feel knowing that someone could do that to you?

What do you think about your survival skills now? Pretty awesome right?

CHAPTER 13 KEEP THE CHANGE

How Intervention Saved My Life

Sometimes when a door closes a better one opens

-Echo Pelster

Thoughts are things, if you can hold them in your mind, you can hold them in your hand- Bob Proctor.

I was glad to be a business owner and involved in the community, but I was still overspending, and still overweight, I was 357.8 pounds in the year 2000, my grandmother died that year and I gained another 20 pounds or so after her death, I did not understand how to deal with grief and death it was overwhelming for me and being an empath I took on the feelings and hurt of others unconsciously through it.

I had been in a grieving stage since I was around 7 years old when my grandfather died getting a drink of water in the night, I learned to fear death when I was very young. I did not know that it was an underlying symptom of my compulsive eating at the time.

Anytime a tear came out of me my mother told me to suck it up and get over it, quit being a ball baby, I remember I must have been 5 years old watching The Wizard of Oz and Dorothy was lost from her Auntie M, I was moved and tearful, my mother made fun of me, I learned that feelings were not acceptable, hide them, bury them, but never show them, if you did there was something wrong with you and it made you weak.

In truth, it made me human, but it would be years before I knew and understood that, and honestly, I had the unreal expectation that my own children should not cry because of this passed down belief, unless they were bleeding of course! Luckily my own pain made me seek better answers, I wasn't perfect, but the timing was perfect, and I could start changing what I could. There really are not any mistakes in the world we will always get what we need when we need it if we are always looking for it. Learn to be a looker.

What a Ludacris way to raise children, what a way to believe as an adult! Feelings run through us all day every day, awake and asleep. They are normal and powerful, and they are manageable, denying them left me wide open to lots of things worse than feelings, it left me open to bad relationships, anorexia, binge eating, no confidence, abused by men sexually and I was not able to trust that having feelings was normal, and when feelings came up I did not know how to respond to them in a healthy way, I pushed them down and out with food, men, and eventually excuses when I had nothing left.

It was when I acknowledged my emotions that I could master them. Feeling and moving through them without reacting to anything or anybody, at least most of the time.

I had left my mother's house and I was still blaming her for the choices and lack of alignment to my own goals here now today, the stories I told myself weren't working anymore.

Mother was wrong in all that happened, but that was hers, now I had to belly up and face my own shortcomings and get on with things.

Whatever I became willing to acknowledge I could overcome. So don't be hard on yourself if you lose your temper, or eat badly for a few minutes, acknowledge it, evaluate what happened, how you can make a better decision next time in a similar circumstance, and move on.

When my brother died, I was nine, and so impressionable and truly believing that because I told him I hated him and because he chased my dog, my dog killed him, my parents then killed my dog Bucky, I was a bad evil little girl for all of their decisions, I was not bad, I was not evil, I lived with people who obviously were, I had done nothing wrong, I learned to speak kinder as a result, and I still do not eat oatmeal. At one point I binged on oatmeal cookies, Joe's death and my choice of oatmeal cookies was the connection. Once I knew the truth, I no longer needed to do that to myself. Always seek the truth.

That was a belief I believed through the treatment and abuse of others. It was not true, it did happen, but I did not have the power to create the result, I was a little girl who argued with a sibling and went to school, whatever happened before I came home that day happened. I am sorry for that, but I did not cause it, create it, or allow it.

When I was 22 my 4th down sister from me died, she was 18, when she died on August 1, 1982, She had been in a coma for two and a half years after being hit by a drunk driver, I never saw her after the accident and I was not at the funeral, mother had moved back to Missouri and every time I wanted to go and see her mother had a reason why I needed to stay away.

Those kids were out on a freezing rain type of night, hit by other kids that were out drinking and partying, my sister's boyfriend was killed instantly that night and my sister lingered, I felt guilty for not having a backbone and making mom let me see her but she was a minor and mom was in control again, I never was able to say goodbye while she still had breathed, I finally went to her grave and said what I needed to say when I was completing my own incompletes. I realize now that because I never saw her in that paralyzed comatose state, I am probably the only person alive that remembers her as she truly was before that car accident. I have learned to look for the good in the most terrible of situations.

She was buried beside her boyfriend that had died two and a half years earlier. I had heard that if that wreck had happened a half-hour earlier all my sisters would have been in that car, as they had all gone roller skating that night, I am grateful that time intervened, even though they are not a part of my life, they rejected me, I am an awesome person and I do not want anything bad to happen to them.

I found out she had died from a stepsister who lived up the street and stood outside yelling your sister is dead! Your sister is dead, until I came out of the house, I was mortified all the neighbors were outside by now, and I did not want anyone to ever know that my mother had married us into this bunch of people, my cover was blown, and yes, my sister was dead and buried by the time I knew she was even dead.

I was hurt, angry, disgusted, and in disbelief at how I found out, and then I settled down, It wasn't what was I thinking, I knew I could not control other people, had someone not told me how would I of even known she was dead, I became grateful for the message and then I could be, and I was the one who believed in treating others like human beings, it hadn't happened before that by my family members, why would I expect anything else now? Because I always had hopes for them that they didn't have for themselves. I still do.

What was I thinking, it was wishing, not real life? Real life in my family had no manners, no etiquette, and milk of human kindness, that's the kind of thing a little girl like me saw in The Wizard of Oz, Gone with the Wind, and Dr. Zhivago, but not in my house, it was a wish, a hope, a desire, and not having it left me an easy target to many predators because I could not tell good from bad, one day something was wrong, the next okay, the unpredictable life I lived as a child left me restless, fearful, discontent, abusive to myself and others at times, and without confidence. It was not who I was, it was who I was to survive, I actually acted out in the play of life, it was not the real me. But until I knew who she was and liked her, I had a fear you wouldn't like her either. I was wrong about that; I like her and so do you. I know because you are still here 12 chapters later.

What was wrong in someone else's home was right in ours, my mother lit my first cigarette for me I was nine, introduced the first man at 12, you get the picture, but I changed the movie when I went places I was uncomfortable, but I was quick to learn, I waited for others to begin eating before I picked up the first fork at a fancy dinner, if I was doing it incorrectly, at least I was doing it incorrectly with everyone else with no judgment, to this day I don't really know which silverware is first, I do know lots of other people don't know either and its ok to follow your hosts lead as long as it is your personal value.

My Sister #8 from me, died on Martin Luther King Day 1995, with twin neighbor boys. I am not sure what truly happened because the truth was always hard to find, one sister told me she was working in the emergency room that day and witnesses told her the kids had been playing chicken with semi's on one-lane bridges around Gorin, Missouri, I don't know if that is true or not, all I know is they were all dead, I decided it was my sister who died who was younger than my oldest son, and I would attend this funeral, I would be there, I would go, to my sisters funeral, I was not at Joe's or Jewel's, I would go to Tonya's no matter what the circumstances, My sister next down that had been in the emergency room, that same sister threatened to beat my ass for showing up, I stood up for myself for the first time and told her if she thought she could we better go outside like ladies, she backed off and that was the end of that, she retreated to her corner, I didn't stay long, but I showed up. I stayed and attended the funeral with my grandparents before going home.

It felt good to muster up the courage and do what I believed was right. Right for me, not dictated by them.

That same year, my mother got to bury another husband. Two holidays in one year, ironically Sister #8 who had died on Martin Luther King's day, her father died on Thanksgiving Day 1995; for some reason we all needed to make it home for Thanksgiving, I arrived the night before, and I went to see this man who persuaded my mother quite easily to give me to the state of Nebraska because I didn't like him, I remember walking out on the front porch that Wednesday night and telling another sister he'll be dead by tomorrow and it won't be natural, but I am sure to someone it will be justifiable. Sure, enough by 1 pm on Thanksgiving Day 1995, he was dead, a few hours later when we returned to that house, everything the man owned was burning in the back of the house, even the bed he slept in, all gone if there was anything to know about the ordeal it was gone, they burned his stuff.

I had no kind words for this man before his death, no it's okay I forgive you for making my life more hell than usual, no pity, no empathy, he was apologizing for what and how he was, I suppose because of some belief he has about himself, or his hereafter. I felt pity for him, I realized he was the one suffering in conscious all of these years, not me, a fascinating reality of acknowledging my own freedom had come and I hadn't recognized it until that day and that moment.

I don't think it mattered. I was simply amused, they put him in a casket and raved about how good he looked, I thought he was dead, and they are still looking at how someone looks and judging the appearance, body image in the casket even. I am amused by the content the world gives me even in such vicarious situations. And as you can see, I write about what you teach me world.

His own kids didn't show up as I remember but I was summoned, I thought what the hell am I supposed to be learning from this? I had no idea, that this last event on the stage was for the people putting it on, not the people who suffered at their hands. It was a relief for their conscious, it was not helpful or useful to me except to know what I didn't want to do, act like or be like in my life. So, it was helpful to know that.

Each time my mother told the story about how stepfather #3 died that day, it was different, not the first time that had happened with a dead husband, as usual, I believe this man was dead. How that happened depends on who you ask, and when the questions are asked, the answer is always different.

I had started to make light of the drama in my mother's house because the Dharma was so dark, no one was fooled, everybody knew, there was no one left to play the game, I didn't eat there, I liked living I decided, and the woman could not be trusted, grandma always said I sure don't want your mom taking care of me, my response, she never has taken care of us, grandma, I don't think she is going to start anytime soon, the care she was talking about was not spelled L-O-V-E it was the kind of care that was not friendly, I DON'T WANT HER TO TAKE CARE OF ME! She was serious. I learned that if I was willing to listen to other people, I could hear the truth, God talks to me through others today, I am grateful for sound answers and the choice of eating the fish and spitting out the bones.

"The only reason people have such a fear of death is that they know nothing beyond the body" -Sadguru

Suicide is a permanent solution to life's temporary, ever-changing problems and conditions, whether it be emotional or real. Our feelings change quickly and often, we do not need to overreact quickly about anything, think it all the way through, then make choices and live well!

And my sister who came to Nebraska and stepped in front of a train, died July 22, 1996, I learned more about powerlessness over the choices of other people than in any other event in my life, I was always powerless, but until I knew it I could not leverage that power. I have learned to surrender and have more control than I could have had by trying to be in control.

My Grandfather who I loved and adored died in November 1997 he had a short illness, he died of an infection he got from the hospital, he should have survived but the MRSA killed him, and I did not see him before he left and transitioned, but I have never felt like he was really gone, just off riding his horse somewhere nearby. I grew up and was not overwhelmed by transition but embrace it today.

Grandma followed Grandpa in October 2000. She and I had always talked about her days being numbered, she called me on my 40th birthday in the year 2000, yes do that math.

We talked for quite a while, she had been living with my sister but now that she was about out of money my sister had slapped her in a rest home, she wanted to go back to Dumas, maybe put a trailer on the right of way near the railroad tracks, she said she thought she had enough left to do that.

I was sad about it all, I knew my sister only took care of her because they wanted her money, when grandma had her stroke and was in the care home recovering, my sister said those words to me personally, and I tried to get others attention, no one listened, the assets were gone, my sister and her husband took it all, but from where I sit karma has kicked in. I do not have to react to anything, anytime, time takes care of every deed, good or bad.

My grandmother was kind and generous to those who were kind to her. She loved her family. She made the best of what she couldn't control, never in my wildest dreams when I talked to her on my birthday October 1, 2000, would I think she would have returned to my sister's house again, only to pass away seven days later, she was blessed with passing away during her morning nap, I am grateful she had an easy transition, she did, and I will always cherish that last birthday card, the one constant throughout my life, and that last phone call, and her saying remember I love you, my dear Echo, you were always the #1 granddaughter, always a sweetie pie.

Grandma always promised to save me a good place on the other side, wherever that was, so after I accomplish being the oldest woman ever recorded in history, I will meet her and the others over there. For me, the biblical heaven came at too high of a cost. I believe everything I was taught actually makes sense for me. I look around and I see God everywhere, just like my grandma did. Life is good, it is all good.

It was a long string of bodies and tragedy. Grandma and Grandpa were the glue that pulled the family together from time to time. After they were gone so were the holidays and going home, I married Vern in 1997 and my grandparents and Aunt Mary loved him, my mother met him at my sister's funeral, and she didn't like him right off because of him being a sheriff's supervisor. I didn't know it then, but he was the good thing that came out of Dell's suicide, it was her idea.

He was a sheriff's deputy supervisor with the Dawson County Sheriff's office where my sister worked, in fact, the Sherriff and all officers of her shift stood graveside to her casket as pallbearers at her funeral. If my mother would have had her way my sister would not have had a funeral, she would have skipped it. I wrote the eulogy and spoke at her funeral; I had found my voice and I had something to say. My speaking career officially started that day I think, if you can speak under the pressure and emotions of suicide you can speak anywhere and do anything.

After my sister's funeral in 1996, my mother being her perfect self said exactly, that she never expected anything less than a suicide from my sister, after all that was how her father died, or did, he? That statement made me realize how I could never change anyone except myself. A leopard does not change its spots, you can't teach an old dog new tricks, but they can desire to learn and teach themselves differently if they want to, but I am powerless over the decisions of other people.

Vern stood there with the other officers that came to my grandparents after the funeral in disbelief, he said to my mother you knew your child was in danger and did nothing, and she was like do what?

Vern told me later he didn't like her attitude either, he tends to stay away from vipers! I totally respect my husband's care and ability to look at and access a situation for what it is. The man has an uncanny ability to think his choices all the way through. Something I have been blessed with the ability to learn and you can too.

About six months after I had met Vern at my sister's funeral I ran into him in downtown Lexington, he asked me what I was doing for Thanksgiving, and I said nothing, my daughter had been married about a year or so and my son was in Oklahoma I think, I said to him why don't we go on a date first, and we've been dating ever since.

As horrible and traumatic as my sister's suicide was I was relieved to find my soulmate in that mess, our 25-year marriage is proof that you have to look for the good in the bad of this life and if you're willing to look for the good you will find it, but I want to tell you if you only go around looking for the bad things in life you will find them also. You can choose the Good.

That is truly the law of attraction we attract into our life who we are, the more confident, the more grateful, and the more blessed we are, and the more appreciative we are for our lives the more we are appreciated. What we give out we receive back every time.

Vern and I lived in a little house when we got married, he had purchased the house nine years before when he was divorced, and he had in 11 year old son, all my friends said you will regret a step child, I never did he was a great kid, but he was a kid and sometime kids have to learn for themselves, I did and I am sure you did to, when I married Vern I did not intend to take his last name, I had worked too restore my own identity and hard to get my name Echo Laymon back, I finally had my own identity and because I had had such rotten luck at marriage prior, I was concerned that if it didn't work out I would have to do all the paperwork to take my maiden name back once again, not much faith in that thought I know, but all the guys in my life were real gents until we were officially married and then the other shoe dropped, but not this time, so when his son came to me and said to me, you know if you take my dad's last name I won't have to explain anything anymore, you know my mom has 3 husbands and us kids all have different names, but if you take my dad's name and be a Pelster then we can just be a family and I don't have to explain anything about that stuff, and the kids anymore, I knew how he felt and I became Echo Pelster when I married LaVern. He is still a great kid today, and we enjoy him and his family whenever possible.

Thoughts are happening all the time. They are emotions, attitudes, health, and behavior, the subconscious mind never sleeps, it stores every word, thought, and picture and the images are acted out based on the underlying belief and the values under those true or untrue beliefs that underpin everything we do.

That's why doing your tomorrow list tonight is such a good thing, because when you do that, your conscious brain sleeps, and your subconscious works out your tomorrow while you sleep.

As a child I was told I was stupid, ignorant, and slow, so that became my performance, only because I believed what I was told. I flunked Mr. Lemons' test for the alphabet and counting because no one had ever taught me how. Once someone taught me, I was able to easily learn, at my house, I was expected to know without being taught so on top of the lack of help and learning, there was giving up trying because I was always wrong no matter what. I was compared to other children which was an insult because I wasn't supposed to be like or as good as someone else, I was supposed to be me. I have learned to make lemons into lemonade. I am smart and resourceful; my resilience is amazing!

And to this day I cannot ever remember anyone being proud of me except my grandparents, my husband, my children, and my sweet loving Aunt Mary. Everyone should have an Aunt Mary. She sees things as experiences, what you do with the knowledge is up to you.

I watched from a distance as the lifestyle killed my siblings one at a time in tragic accidents and suicides, after a while, there was no amount of anything that could make me feel better. I could eat a swimming pool of twinkies and not feel better, I am grateful I couldn't, because I heard her and this time I responded to her differently, I gave her what she had been calling for all along, I wrote her, I saw her, I became her, I was grateful to cope with life through binge eating and food were how I coped something had to give. Awareness was the power that saved my life.

Grandma and grandpa loved me but the message I remember was them being disappointed about my choices and the directions I took, but I am not sure they weren't proud of me, because most people were critical that criticism stayed with me for a long time. I had to approve of myself to recognize their approval. Their generosity and their gifts supported me when I aligned on a better life path.

My grandfather quit celebrating my birthday because I dropped out of school and got pregnant, I am sure now he was disappointed in my choices, I did the predicted, mom was proud of my life being ruined and my grandparents were worried for me and the next generation, rightfully so, but it felt like at the time he didn't love me anymore. He did he loved me and protected my heart. He understood me and cared with great intention.

I craved approval and I realized he did love me very much and he understood how soft-hearted I was, when after my sister's suicide, he waited a week to personally call me which was something he had never done, to tell me my aunt had died, my grandma Echo's sister, he told me it was just too much too soon after my sister's death and suicide. He knew it would hurt me, but for 23 years I heard he didn't love me in my head because of the birthday thing, and then I heard he did. Reprogramming is a tedious job.

QUESTIONS TO ASK YOURSELF & JOURNAL ABOUT:

Do you blame anyone for a family members death? Is it true?

How do you know?

Did you ever ask for an investigation? Why or why not?

Were you embarrassed, was there blame, or shamed into being quiet?

If so, how does that fear still affect you? Why? How have you dealt with the event till now?

Do you tell people about your family?

Are you proud of who you are and where you come from? What are you most afraid people would think if they knew?

What are you most afraid of feeling if others knew family secrets? Has me telling the secrets that freed me, been valuable to you?

How has it helped?

What do you see more clearly now? How will that help you in the future?

Are you excited to know that freedom is a choice?

CHAPTER 14

Releasing the Pounds of Pain

"Never love something so much that you can't let go of it" - unknown

&

The Next Attempt to Release the Pounds of Pain

"Surrender is what is, let go of what was, have faith in what will be."
Sonia Ricotti

When I couldn't take it anymore, I just stopped in my tracks, in 2001 I was diagnosed with congestive heart failure, and weighed 358 pounds! I couldn't walk up the stairs in my house without stopping several times, I could hardly get dressed without being out of breath, and still, the compulsion to eat was screaming from inside me, no matter what my intention was to take care of myself and eat right I could not. I was no longer in control of it, it was in control of me.

I was like every dieter who heard the voice of a thin friend say you must stay on your weight loss program, your diet, no matter what you must discipline yourself, just do it!

Well, friends, there is no "PERFECT DIET" for this problem, we know what to eat and what not to eat. Our eating is a profound rejection of ourselves. It is a moment of betrayal and self-punishment. Anything but the commitment to one's well-being, why would anyone think we could commit to a diet of any kind, if you're not already committed to yourself.?

So, I stopped dieting and lost over 100 pounds! Once I discovered that my relationship with food reflected my relationship with myself, I placed my loyalty in my love for myself.

Self-hate was acted on by putting all the non-food food items in my body, always unconsciously to cover up a feeling or some uncomfortable painful memories or events. Self-hate foods were always high-density sugary fat producing foods. Foods that destroy.

Self-Love came when I chose to move through the uncomfortable painful memories or events. Then I could decide to eat real food items and make good decisions for myself every time. Self-love foods were always life-giving foods, God's foods, Served his way. Foods that heal.

This was after my first gastric stapling in 1984, trying to be thin enough, loveable enough, beautiful enough, I was always looking for the answers outside of myself, I only weighed 224 pounds when I had that first gastric procedure, what happened? The truth was my inner self was calling, calling me to notice and love me, I did, I gave her a bariatric stapling procedure. It soothed her for a little while, and then her self-loathing demanded attention and ate and ate.

I lost down to about 160 and then something happened, and I started gaining again, I coped with food, all my sense of love and peace was around food, every single day I got up with the intention of eating right and exercising and every afternoon I and my friend Little Debbie, Snickers and the gang got together and blew it. My friends were massive criminals that kept me isolated and hiding out! Lets look at their street names.

Lays a name for a potato that also brings shame if you lay with too many people. Shame producing.

Snickers, laughs at you, and makes fun of you! bullied you, and makes you feel bad about yourself.

Cookie, something you are supposed to be for everyone. Little Debbie, a name from a bad porn show.

They all were names that made me feel like and imposter every time we got together. I had to give up who I hung out with at home and come out of isolation. I had to get a batch of new friends and leave the alone zone forever.

I had done every diet in the book and then it occurred to me to do another gastric bypass, never mind that the first one nearly killed me, and I was in the hospital for 6 weeks with an infection.

I only lost 60 pounds and later gained clear upto 357.8 pounds over the next few years, what the heck let's do it again! Crazy is an understatement, insane is probably closer! So I had another Gastric By-pass, this time a Roux N Y, I lost 203 pounds, I was honored by a huge article in the local paper, only to gain back almost 114 pounds, I had gone from proud of myself to hiding out and isolating, all my old friends were back in the house, and heroin has the same characteristics as sugar, white powders are white powders, my drug of choice was sugar, destructive to my teeth and my body.

I went to work and home, I was so ashamed, I didn't understand why I continued to sabotage myself with the secret eating and the consumption of sometimes more than 20,000 sugar calories in an evening, I felt sick, but I couldn't stop myself.

It wasn't the food I was eating it was my spirit.

It wasn't what I was eating, it was what was eating me.

After the gastric Roux N Y, I had plastic surgery to remove all the skin, I was so embarrassed, I didn't understand why I couldn't just quit. I feared the idea of giving up what gave me comfort, but it didn't give me comfort, it gave me pain, a lot of pain. Self-judgment, self-criticism, and self-loathing is all pain.

Why did I run back? Because I had failed to replace the painful past with present love and a fearless future. The fact was God was committed to me but I didn't find myself worth it. This was part of his divine plan for me, life is programmed for the highest level of creativity and good. Helping others get what they want has helped me get what I want.

Sugar was my Nemesis and I needed to part with it forever. Or so I believed.

So, I was spiritually ill, but I had been in church my whole life, how does that happen. Oh, You too? It's because we become what we hide. And my binge eating was a secret, or at least I thought it was, really? It was hanging all over me. All over my body.

I realized I had an addiction, and I decided to try some support groups, but they were alcoholics and laughed at me because even open groups didn't consider something like sugar addiction real, but it was and is for many people, especially if they have used it to replace, love, joy, kindness, and nurturing that they haven't learned to separate the emotions from the feeling of feeling better.

The relief was always what I was looking for. It was only a momentary bliss, an illusion. I realized loneliness played a part, but how could that be, I was around people all day long at work, came home to a family, and still ate secretly.

My surgeon retired and the doctor who took his place turned out not to be a plastic surgeon at all.

QUESTIONS TO ASK & JOURNAL ABOUT FOR YOURSELF:

What do you binge on? What is your guilt like?

How many family dinners did you go to and hardly eat a thing?

How many times did you go home and binge because of those dinners?

How do you associate food to love?

What foods show the most love for you and your body? What food show the most pain for you heart and body?

What is a food that you know should be a below the line food for you?

CHAPTER 15

If I feel my Emotions I will fall apart.
Barbie is plastic, I am not

"Our greatest glory is not in never failing, but in rising up every time we fail"- Ralph Waldo Emerson

After my abdominoplasty went so well, I wanted to have the skin removed from my arms and legs. But the original doctor had moved away, and I truly considered going to Louisiana where he had moved for the sake of his family, his kids were having a hard time in a rural school in western Nebraska, I had spoken to him, but he felt I would need to stay in the south for a few weeks as it was a pretty big surgery and it just became too expensive of an idea.

I went to the other plastic surgeon, and something didn't feel right but I wasn't listening to my gut. First, what doctor comes out to meet the patient and take them back to the patient's room? Red Flag! #1

Everywhere else in the world was a nurse doing this. I had asked my gastric surgeon if he thought he was any good. He said yes, so I trusted his referral. And scheduled the surgery. It was April 10, 2010, the cost was over 10,000 dollars all out-of-pocket expenses as it was again elective, I expected a 7-inch incision under my arms and about 12 inches in my inner thighs. And a small incision at the edge of each breast to remove a sack area of skin on each side, a procedure that takes normally 2 hours, I was in surgery for more than 7 hours, I was cut from my knee to my groin, and on both sides of my groin, there were no hidden tiny stitches but big ugly staples, Nearly 1500 of them, the surgeon was a man named Nissan Byatt, I had staples all the way across my chest and from my wrists to my armpits I looked like Frankenstein's monster.

Over 1500 awful big ugly staples, he informed me after the surgery that he decided to change the plan and he decided to give me some bonuses for the surgical work I did not pay for, in addition, he did the groin work so I could have more sexual pleasure, I felt instantly sexually violated and told him to get out of my room. He was full of explanations why, but they were all excuses, the surgery nurses came to my room and said I should protect myself with legal counsel, I reached out to hospital administration immediately.

Bound in bandages from head to toe, I told my little 7-month pregnant nurse that I had horrible pain in my right arm, I had mentioned it in recovery, several times, she called the doctor and he said she was fine and he went home, the next day I complained about the arm again, I felt like my skin was going to bust, that night it did, I almost bled to death, a priest gave last rights, on the way to surgery in the elevator, for the life of me, I guess I was really scared. The next morning, I woke to a 47,000-dollar out-of-pocket medical bill.

I had already made a formal complaint to the administration before almost bleeding to death about him enhancing my sexual pleasure, how dare he cut and violate me this way!

I signed for plastic surgery, with no scars, or at least minimal and he violated me by doing procedures and assuming I would like them without my signature and approval, and I knew it.

The first time they got me out of bed the next day my legs started bleeding and oozing everywhere spilling out on the carpet.

He noticed a high sed rate and put me on an antibiotic, and sent me home, every day I felt worse, I kept calling and no response from the great doctor N. B., who by now turned out not to be a certified plastic surgeon at all. Finally, I called a local physician at his home at 5 am, I was sick, and I knew it. He gave me two shots of Rocephin and saw me again the next day, gave me two more, and on the third day, I called my gastric surgeon and headed back to the Regional medical center.

When we arrived, they saw that all 6 JP tubes were running white, I was septic, and I told my trusted gastric surgeon not to let that crazy Bayat near me, I was admitted and isolated immediately.

I was in extreme pain, with a 104 fever and extremely high MRSA count, I extremely wanted this doctor by the neck now, I was so angry, he was ordered by the hospital to stay away from me.

During the night the next night, I woke up and Dr. N.B. was standing at the end of my bed at about 2 am. I was horrified, he was obviously under the influence of something, he was crying, asking me not to sue him, and holding a needle with something in it in his hand. The nurse had taped the nurse call to my hand earlier because I could hardly move, I pressed the button and held it with everything I had because I did not want her to talk through the intercom I wanted her to come, to come now and to come quickly, they came running into the room and the doctor ran out, then I was moved immediately, the hospital continued to move me around to keep me safe for the next few weeks, finally Bayat was suspended, removed by security and I was safe. Or at least told I was.

I spoke to a lawyer once I was home, it had been ten weeks and I still was not well, but I was down to 150 pounds, what a way to lose weight, almost dying, now with horrible scars, and on top of it C- Diff, Mono, it was a long 6 months, in order to sue this idiot doctor I was informed that I would also have to sue the guy who saved my life also, laws are totally screwed up in the malpractice world, and I could not do that, my insurance did kick in after 24 hours and if I won a malpractice suite I would have to pay back everything insurance had paid, I had the risk of not getting enough in a settlement to cover it all as the bills now totaled over 200,000 dollars.

I couldn't bring suit against the people who saved my life it was against my own integrity. But I could tell the world about that crappy surgeon who was moving from state to state, hospital to hospital pretending to be a plastic surgeon I could tell and hopefully save other American women from being violated by this pretender. I forgive his incompetence, I would probably forgive it even more with a refund, and compensation for wearing long sleeves since 2010.

Since he left Nebraska, by the way, he was a general surgeon in Michigan before Nebraska, then he went to Boston Massachusetts, then to California, and last I heard he was in Texas.

After my ordeal he threatened to sue and sued the regional medical center, I got the call, after everything that happened the hospital wrote off all my out-of-pocket bills, so of course, when I was asked to testify against Dr. N.B., I said yes, I told them I would take my clothes off for a jury if necessary. My scars were hideous, and they still are, he left me butchered and ashamed to wear a sleeveless dress or top. After I worked so hard to lose the weight, I took my anger of what he had done out on myself, unconsciously of course, I was angry at me for trusting him.

I must have something wrong with me if I could trust an imposter like that!

I have spent the last 12 years wearing long sleeves to hide the hideous scars that the butcher left me with, he cut my perspiration glands, the antibiotics left me with systemic alopecia on my arms, and the emotional pain and abuse Dr. B inflicted have been traumatic, to say the least, and the least he could have done was offer me a refund, oh, that might be admitting wrongdoing on his part, but I think KARMA is in charge, I trust it is, he could admit he was wrong and settle through his malpractice insurance, it would have at least left himself with some honor.

But I decided he must not have any and if he is practicing it is important to tell my story for the sake of every person that could accidentally seek out his services, the fancy office looks inviting. But there is a reason why a waiting room is empty.

Dr. N.B. dropped the lawsuit against the Nebraska medical center once he knew I was testifying. He proved to be self-preserving because I knew if he lost there, I would get another shot at him in a courtroom, apparently, he did too.

Devastated emotionally, physically and still somewhat in shock from being victimized by this doctor, I was gaining weight a few pounds each month, It felt crazy, I had no reason to stay thin and healthy with these scars, I couldn't even look at my body, one leg still has a whole, the infections caused the staples to rot out of my skin, they tore away as a slimy mess, for months and months staples worked out of my skin for about 3 years. But this time I was realizing something.

I had plenty of warning signs about this guy and I wasn't listening to my own inner voice, my intuition. I realized I could have avoided him if my own self-love was more than plastic acceptance of myself.

Again, I had looked outside myself for the answers that were inside, I heard the little voice, faint as it was saying no, no, no, and I didn't trust it, and I was butchered because of that. I accept my part in it, it does not make his butchery acceptable.

He was wrong, he more than likely should have never chosen to do my surgery, I suspect he knew he was not qualified! But he also maybe should have read Psycho-Cybernetics by Dr. Maxwell Maltz.

I finally left the private support groups, they were their own kind of religion or cult of sorts, and then I tried going back to religion, and that was definitely not bringing back any peace and then I started reading everything I could on food addiction until I found some principles that not only work for me but will work for anyone who applies them, I tried programs developed by Tony Robbins and other famous people, but they were more of a fad, not a lifestyle.

Although I love Tony, I met him in Omaha Nebraska before he was famous, he was a tall skinny kid really selling VHS tapes and cassettes of his weight loss program, I remember telling him I had no idea what skinny people eat, and he said everything, just not so much of it.

There was good information, but I knew it had to be a way in which no one was controlling how much and what kinds of foods I was eating, I had to have all the food I needed, and I even had to change my definition of what real food was, was it food or chemical, toxic waste? Once I developed a module to learn that that would be individualized for everyone who would try my program,

I realized I was on to some concepts that would work for individuals based on their own values about food.

I started biohacking food and its sources, molds, contamination, and the names of sugar which now has nearly 100 deceptive names for sugar on food labels, so unless you are up on it you are eating sugar and not even aware of it, and the fact that most natural flavors are artificial chemicals to enhance your taste buds and make you want more of their food brands is totally another book.

I had to stop eating unconsciously, and I needed structure, I didn't know how to decipher all the millions of food information and theory's available, I looked at famous hospital diet plans, but that was where people went because they were sick, I wasn't sick again not yet, I kept my exercise and walking each day up even when I returned to eating poorly.

Eating often is never anyone's problem, it's eating poorly often that is a problem, because it is self-hate. Eating well often is a form of self-love.

I drink a large amount of water, coffee, and tea, I like herbal cleansing teas or fruit teas, no sugar of course in the evening, some teas are inspirational, read the box and see what resonates with you.

Fruits, Vegetables, and Unprocessed Meat is my friend today, Chemicals and Sugars are below-the-line foods for me today. Chemicals because if I cannot pronounce them, they should not be in my body, Sugars because I am a self-proclaimed sugar addict. What starts out as a little becomes a lot, and even a lot is not enough. So I choose not to go there, not to go through it anymore, not to punish myself that way, I chose to love myself today.

Deep Breathing and Relaxation Techniques reduce your cortisol levels naturally and meditation renews your heart, mind, and intuition. Conscious Contact with a power greater than myself leads me to the best love, best satisfaction, the best peace.

So, I started out by increasing my fluid intake, deep breathing, and meditation, I started looking inside for the answers to my life, they were never outside of me, they were never separate from me, we are taught to look outside ourselves for everything today by the person selling the next best thing. We don't need to I had every single ingredient I needed, and you do too.

Since I already didn't eat gluten because of gluten intolerance and it was the same for dairy due to lactose intolerance, but on a binge, I might do it all and make myself sick for days. It was cunning and baffling. Often, I would come out of a binge with a big what just happened after having a few clean weeks or months, and I didn't understand why.

I knew deep down the problem was sugar and I started biohacking sugar and realized it was my nemesis, sugar had to go, all sugar, sugar substitutes, everything, the first week was literally the shits, I mean diarrhea, upset stomach, headache, dehydration, all of everything that people talked about with drug and alcohol addiction. It was awful, but I knew there would be an end.

Even artificial sugars taste sweet and set off the insulin response, not to mention what they are made of, look at that and then look where that comes from. Nope, I am not putting that in my brain.

I have learned since that sugar is 30 times more addictive than heroin and in everything, it's 40% of the average bottle of ketchup, which I loved, it's in pasta sauce, and of course, pasta and all other grains convert to sugar in the body and make the sugar addict want more sugar.

I had to make some serious lifestyle changes, but it's been worth it,

I know what you are thinking, like where do you get your calcium without milk, and your brain needs carbohydrates, I will say yes, they do, however, I will also tell you that the country's like Sweden and England who drink the most milk have the highest rates of osteoporosis, Prostate, and ovarian cancer.

Leafy greens will provide lots of calcium also like spinach and kale, I have a big green shake of those every day now.

I learned all the different types of hunger, and that treats may be mistreating me. Don't listen to your head, listen to your hunger, real hunger. I eat nothing that is bad for me in moderation, if it is something I need to moderate I need to have moderate health with it. I don't want moderate health, so I don't want it. Whatever it is, not even once in a while, I love myself enough to make that decision today.

I truly believe the food manufacturers put a lot of sugar in things because they know how addictive it is, and you will eat more than you need and buy more food and it lines their pockets very nicely because today if I get a little sugar in something I am not expecting I always think it tastes gross.

When you feed your sugar habit the habit screams for more sugar, starve it and it goes away!

Today I recognize hunger from thirst, variety from boredom, the food angels in my head that say oh, you have been so good, and the food devils that say oh, just a little won't hurt you, I recognize how being too hungry, lonely, tired, or angry can affect me, I practice gratefulness and live here, now in this day presently.

I hold no resentments as they are like throwing my own life to the wind. I live and let live. Like I said it wasn't what I was eating it was what was eating me.

I learned that people were sad to see me gain again, but they were also on my side. I no longer isolate myself; I get involved and take part. Help someone else, anything, I don't buy non-food items, no excuses to bring them home like they are for the dog or the grandkids, no they are hardly ever here if I buy that crap, I will eat that crap, I will own that responsibility right now!

If I buy it it's because I am planning a binge and I am going to eat it eventually in a bad moment if it is available when that bad moment comes, not having it in the house will never stop anyone who is planning a binge, there are lots of grocery stores and restaurants, but it may give you the opportunity to stop yourself, call a friend or work your own program out with a coach, if it's not too handy.

I no longer chose to allow any event or circumstances to derail my love for myself, I respond differently, in a beneficial way, sometimes I just wait, feelings change quickly. I try to never re-act to anything, but at the appropriate time respond.

Sometimes I write or read something, I meditate, and I care about myself today. I always connect to the source, which I call God or the Universe simultaneously, to me it's the same thing, it's the magic power greater than myself, the secret sauce.

The way I get through each challenge is to ask myself what the next right move is, and then the next, and then the next, because my life is not defined by one moment. Sometimes I just breathe through the moment and do nothing, I notice my thoughts, are they my thoughts or something I was once told, I listen through my true self instead of my ego self today.

By giving myself clear, strong healthy redirection, changing every negative into a positive when I am conscious enough to catch it, consciousness is looking to the power that I call God and listening to the answers that I believe come from that great universal power, not separate from me, but within me, I have changed my life. Let's talk about how you can change yours also.

My business was failing due to a local manufacturing plant closing in our area, most of my clients were transferred away within 30 days and I was next up financially, I tried moving my business to a more populated area, but by the end of 3 years we were sinking, the business was breakeven with the 60 customers we had left, and I suddenly could not make a living after 25 years, so I liquidated and moved on, and struggled with my weight and coped with sugar. I realize now that that was God telling me my latter was against the wrong wall, he was pulling me in a new direction.

Everything became easy at that moment since I listened to my inner voice, life has become much easier, my authenticity has surfaced, and my work writing is my passion, like breathing, my energy force is passion. Passion to help those who suffer compulsively.

It is not the role I play today, like a financial advisor, it is my passion for talking about the limitless possibilities that life itself offers, the truth is weight was not my issue, it was my distraction. Weight was what kept me from living life, feeling feelings, enduring pain, and enjoying pleasure. Now I can eat appropriately and live abundantly.

Weight was the distraction that stopped me from looking within, it kept me the people pleaser, and it kept me dependent on the opinions of others, when I had the courage to go within, to hear my own inner voice the weight falls away. Where the mind goes the body follows.

I was food addicted and even though I had, had, 2 gastric bypass surgeries, I was gaining weight again, you can't fix a secret.

Ironically, I applied the principles I had developed and went from a size 30 to a size 12. And I have kept it off for more than 20 years now. This was a belief, not a truth, today I can be around any food and make a conscious decision within that day, in the presence of today if it is right or wrong for me, this is true food freedom, the freedom of choice.

QUESTIONS TO ASK AND JOURNAL ABOUT:

How is my dialogue with food today?

What am I pretending not to know?

Am I ready to get down and really let go of what no longer serves me?

If I let it go, how do I imagine my life without it?

What will you do to fill your time now that you stopped eating? How will you exit the alone zone and never isolate again?

How will you love yourself, appreciate yourself and be kind to yourself today?

How will you do the shadow exercise to get a vision of your thin self?

Wrap your arms around yourself and look in the mirror for 5 minutes today, tell yourself aloud every beautiful thing you see in your eyes, features, and body. How does it feel?

What is food to you now? Does it have a life? Chemicals? Junk? Whatever you decide food is that's what you eat, only that, you will gage your food life around this answer, when you have a special occasion, you will eat only what is real food to you.

How will it be to allow yourself to eat real food and enjoy the event? (that's the real food to you, the list does not change because of the circumstances today.)

Can you honor your decision and trust yourself with this or do you need more help? I trust you I know you know how best to take care of yourself.

Can we start taking down the wall you built around yourself with food now?

Are you ready to remove your big heavy coat and reveal your beautiful self to the world?

Before when you were afraid or anxious you ran to food, what will you do now to take care of yourself, right some good for yourself activities down, plan for life to happen and for you to handle it positively.

Who can you call? Go For a Walk?

Cup of Tea and Relax and Breathe?

What is the color of your next new outfit?

Now that you are no longer camouflaging your body with weight how do you see yourself.?

CHAPTER 16

What I Learned & You can too!

"I learned that people would forget what you said, People will forget what you did, but people will never forget how you made them feel"

–Maya Angelou

This is one of the most important quotes in this book, it is the one that forces me within myself, the one that reminds me how others made me feel, and how I made others feel, it reminds me where I needed to say I am sorry, I was wrong, I want you to be complete, I want me to be complete. It is the quote that brings me to this heart-to-heart.

This was the place I could not come until my own mud was ripe enough that the seed of myself could sprout into the woman I would become, the mud I was raised in is not the fragrance of my life today, but I had to go through the mud to come to the amazing gratefulness of my life and realize the message that came out of those muddy swampy places.

How can you start laying down the past and living in today, you are not there anymore, what do you imagine freedom to look and be like for you?

I had to be ready for the change, ready for the intuition, and intention, ready for the purposeful powerful life I was given in grateful experience.

How do you show your gratitude every day, do you say thank

you, tell others how much you appreciate them, thank yourself for the care you give yourself each day, love yourself?

I had to yield to the inner voice, the voice of calling that is never quiet, to become the one that would represent the tens of thousands.

How will use this information to help someone else? Will you give them a copy of the book? Tell them about the book? Do a book study with others who are asking you about all the noticeable changes in your life? What will you do?

I had to realize the magnitude and become willing to receive the triumph and blessing of every hard moment, every hurt feeling, and every opportunity to renew my spirit.

What are you willing to do today that you have dug your heels in about in the past? Do you need to apologize to someone? Do you need to forgive yourself; can you want others to have the happiness you want for yourself?

I had to realize that there was no more waiting to be loved, I am humbled to know that I am loved. It is within the soft flesh of the oyster that a wound creates a great and beautiful pearl. I AM that pearl.

Can you recognize your wounds as pearls yet? What amazing resilience you have because of your past? Can you love yourself and be gentle with yourself and find yourself precious in your eyes and your chosen creators' eyes?

I had to un hostage myself to the future and not use the past as a weapon toward myself. It was a gift of great opportunity.

Are you ready to set yourself free? Untie the imaginary ropes and false limitations and go after what you really want?

I had to evolve to resolve, heal to reveal, and practice the presence of God within myself, love myself, I could not give to others what I did not possess, I had to forgive myself for what I did not know, I will always try to do better in consciousness now that I know better. I am sorry. I love you. Please forgive me. Thank you. I pray that is enough for those I hurt in the process.

How will you fill yourself up with so much love that you have lots and lots to give away? What are some kind actions and words you will always have available for yourself? Forgive yourself now for what you did not know yesterday, we do better when we know how to do better.

How will you lead by example in the future and love the loveless to heal the hurt you caused others and others caused you? Love anyway.

Today I know I am enough. I had to realize I only lost my power when I gave it to other people, the ego thrives on the opinion of another, it eats the negative words and opinions of another like candy, it sucks the life out of me with the messages of unworthiness and negative beliefs, the ego is rooted in the negative beliefs of us and others, judgments of others closed- mindedness of others and self. I had to give up my ego and its negative opinions of me. I remember every day that the opinion of others about me is none of my business.

How will you keep up your power through perfect surrender to the things that are not in your power to fix each day? How will you set your ego aside so you can do the right thing each time you need to? How will you remember that what other people think of you is none of your business?

The ego loves chaos and pain, the ego lives in the past and the future, not the present. Ego is the fear of another person's approval or opinion.

How will you not worry about what others think of you when you choose the best way to live your life? Raise your family? Provide for your family? Have you given up the disease to please?

I had to learn that the soul lives in the present, Echart Toll taught me to hold my hands 12 inches apart, what is on the outside of the left hand is the past, what is outside the right hand is the future, and what is between them is the present, the soul is rooted in the present, in love when you are perceiving from the soul, not from what you do that is your role in life, your soul is where you live in life in the right now.

How will you keep yourself in today? Let yesterday be a faded memory? An experience you simple learned from? How will you let tomorrow wait until tomorrow? How will you plan without setting and expectation of how you think things should be?

I had to learn that I AM IS THE WAY, only in the presence of God do I access the power of the present moment, in the silence I can access the power of God within me, but I will not let this be a poor substitute or the reality of God. The power of life is God, in the soul of God, there is no judgment. Oneness with this force as I understand it is all life.

How are you starting to see your power? What name will you give it? How will or do you thank it? Gratitude? Love for Yourself and others?

I had to learn that Karma is grace itself, bad karma, bad childhood=grace=surrender. The space where unconditional divine consciousness came into my life, was already there anyway, so I just as well move into it, go with its flow of inspiration at this moment. When I surrendered to it I became strong and felt young again.

How will you accept who you are? Where have you come from? How will you embrace the past as your strength for your future?

I had a choice I could stay in why does this always happen to me, why did it, that would be keeping bad karma, and making more of it, or I could use the bad karma for good, I choose to feel the bad karma when it comes and recognize the feelings and how the experience benefits me.

How will you allow the feelings that run through you every moment of everyday to run through you like a soft stream, feel them and accept them?

I had to realize that no one knows the thought of God, except the spirit of God, I am a person or form, my spirit lives here, I am a part of God and God is a part of me when my body is done, then my spirit will move out of the body. God lives with me in this body, we are a part of each other, God does not kill himself, his own spirit he will not kill me, or anyone else. I did ask him once why he doesn't like sugar, because if I struggle with it, he must also, since he lives here, he laughed and said, Really, I made sugar too. You may change your mind about it someday, I thought will that be justification to fall off the wagon, or get on?

How will you get rid of old ideas that no longer serve you and claim and inspire ideas that will allow you to be happy, joyous and free?

I had to realize that as a child I felt the closeness of God and knowing that I was God's child, but it was shadowed and overcast by the judgments of other people and the actions of my rapist, rape in a young or any person leaves cynicism behind. I was cynical of

God's love because of that man's actions, but God had nothing to do with it, and I did not in any way solicit the bad actions of another, it was not true, in my darkest hour God remained my father, and hell is not offered by my loving God. When we each must choose to do the right thing, God's support will always be there because we made that right choice. My rapist only won if I gave him my mind also.

How will you resolve your past mentally and emotionally in self-preservation?

I had to learn that my internal yearning and calling were the direct connection between me and the entity that I choose to call God today, the part that connects me to my higher self. I was his when I was unwanted, I was a child of convenience, to get my parents from where they were in their young lustful lives to where they wanted to be, but they did not truly want me, I was just the tool of their own freedom, I don't believe they knew I would be hostage, I am still God's child and he gave me a purpose, and it whispers in my heart that they will still someday want to know who I am, they are still living but it hasn't been their desire. But I bask in the light of my true father's love that gives me the strength to do what needs to be done each day in the right light. I will never be able to make people more than they are. They have to choose that journey to their higher self for themselves.

How will you except others for who they are not who you want them to be?

I had to realize that when I was on the wrong path in life was where I had the most unhappiness. Those times when I didn't listen to my gut, my inner voice, and I went anyway. My gut is there to warn me today I listen, it doesn't matter the hour of the day, only that I take the action necessary and listen closely.

How will you trust your own instincts about everything first? Be able to do what's best for you? Take care of yourself with no fear?

I had to learn I don't fail, and I don't lose when I get knocked down, but when I fail to get back up. Often these knockdowns have been God the inner calling me, telling me you are going the wrong way,

I am thankful for those turbulent unhappy, unfulfilling times that allowed me to move on and come here in this now.

How will you recover when you get off course? How will you get back on course? How will you use every challenge for growth and good?

I had to realize that my original and truest nature is reverence for all life, every form, from the leaf or the blade of grass, from the tree to the organism in the pond or the tick on my dog. It is all life, and life force, connected, oneness, with the universe, which I call God.

How will you treat everyone and every living thing kindly?

I had to learn that I will attract into my life who I am, and when I am living at my highest self-others may not be comfortable around me yet, now, or ever, but I will do my absolute best to reveal my highest self with intentional living.

How will you let your light shine even when you are afraid? How will you stay positive when you have anxiety trying new things? How will you trust the process?

I learned that I had to come out of the shadows, the tricky places that the ego takes me, and thrive in the sunlight.

How will you step into the light when there are suddenly clouds that were not in the forecast?

I had to love and respect the dark and allow it, to feel it. So, I could move into the light and enjoy it, bask in it, and embrace it all.

How will you joyfully embrace the simple joy of each day?

I had to learn that there is not a quick fix for my life, sometimes the shadows return, just as I lost my faith as I believed I was rooted into the approval of my mother, I realized that the one thing she really gave me was faith, she sent me off were she thought I could be better off. There is a state of mind that all of us will be challenged with at some point in life, the bigger challenge is to thrive in it and bloom.

How will you turn the lemons into lemonade each day? How will you remember your attitude is your choice?

I had to learn to listen, my sister told me her intention to take her own life months before she did, I did not recognize the acronym in the moment, hindsight is always 20/20, and I am not responsible for the choices of others, I respect her choice of transition, I am sorry it was needed. Such a permanent solution to life's temporary problems.

How will you continue to forgive yourself as memories return that were buried with the past? Will you look it over, or chew on it a while? How will you let it go?

I learned to believe other people when people tell me today who they are, I believe them, their actions, their words, they know themselves better than I know them, I choose to believe them, and I choose to honor requests that are bad for them, I know they must do their own knowing and learning, and I gratefully and graciously push away the people who are the insulters and assaulters of my life and forgive them silently on their way out.

When others show you who they are how will you deal with them? The opportunity to grow is always beautiful, but what if they continue to disrespect or abuse you? Then what?

I remain precious in my own eyes. And in God's, no need to be abused or disrespected ever. Forgiveness for their actions and words yes. Trust must be earned after such events.

How will other be allowed to rebuild trust? When will you say enough is enough? How will you know? How will you stay safe? Are there any people who will never have the privilege of trust? If so who are they so you never forget your why.

I had to learn that when someone showed me who they are to believe them, after my mother gave me a way to the state of Nebraska, I wanted things the way they were before, they never could be, I wanted the abusive neglective life back because I did not know how to live outside the chaos in peace.

How many times is someone allowed to break your heart before you walk away? How will you deal with the uncomfortableness of not being abused? Can you love being loved and cared for? Can you allow yourself the gift of choosing to be happy no matter what the world is doing?

Happiness is the decision we make for ourselves.

After a year of kindness and sorting out all that I had experienced, I went back, and the pain returned, I have hurt repeatedly because of putting myself into the aim of my parents and their justification of my bad treatment, anytime I went back to my immediate family i.e., my mother's house, I cried all the way home and for days after. I always hoped it would be nice this time that they had changed the more I changed the more I realized they hadn't and probably never would I had to accept who they were not who I wanted them to be.

Can you choose not to go where nothing ever changes? Can you always choose to protect yourself and your dignity? No matter what? If you go back to an unhappy place, can you quietly go if needed? Can you do that for yourself?

I had to learn I could change no one except myself. Every time I put my hand back into that cage I was bitten. I have no regrets, but my cup runs over today and there is no longer room for that in my life. Side note: I reached out to my mother some 18 months ago hoping that she would desire to change how her and my story ends. When she answered her phone and heard it was me her reply was "HELL NO". I believed her, thanked her for telling me, and chose not to look back, I have a child who lives in that area, and I am glad to say I can go to him on occasion and not need to even drive by her home. I am finally truly free.

Can you cut your losses and know you are better for them? How can you see the blessings and not the bitterness? How can you be grateful for you life today?

I had to be honest with what I believed and what was always right for me. When I was pregnant as a teenager, I did not love the fathers of my babies and they did not love me. I did not need to marry anyone, all that did was ruin 4 lives because of an idea that I needed to be married if I was having a baby, I did not, I could and should have been allowed to do for my babies what I thought was best for them, no one had the right to force me into a marriage, so there could be enough money to take care of us, the highest self in me believed there would always be enough, it had faith, the ego wanted to please and lived horribly to please and satisfy the opinions of others. The ego is a big fat liar.

How will You do what's best for you in each circumstance? Setting aside the opinions of others and listening to yourself and your higher power?

I learned I must always take care of myself first, or I have nothing to give to others. And be okay with being done with those who hurt you and do you harm, they are done with you when they do this.

How will you embrace yourself and put yourself first when it is needed?

I know that history cannot be unlived, wars cannot be unfought, hurtful words cannot be withdrawn, my weight was only a distraction, the soul is the spirit that longs for all and everything, God is the Soul, it is everywhere, in everything, in me, with me there are so many paths to the place inside, the most revealing path is the silent one for me. Not the praying, petitioning, and begging silence but the quiet waiting, knowing, and hearing that happens in the silence that only I can hear, feel, and partake of. My personal inspiration and life breathe from God.

When I feel like my higher power is far away how will I bring it closer to me? How will I connect with others like me and create new and lasting friendships? How will I stay out of the alone zone?

I had to find myself in the silence, replacing the food with wisdom and love, and recognize my own resilience.

What space will you keep each day to practice silence and meditation for your emotional wellbeing? Prayer? Ritual Studies? Biblical? What fits who you see you being?

I had to realize that for every action there is a reaction, and every single bit of it was for my benefit, I learn daily to embrace it in the present. What may have been intended by others for my harm is for my good, a blessing.

How will you look for the good in every single situation?

I had to learn that my value was not the words others spoke to me in anger or disapproval, are not my worth or value, I am not the definition of any other man or woman, I am the definition of the I AM that is the way. I Am in my own Spirit with my Christ consciousness, I know who I am through his model of how I try to live my life, precious, valued, loved, and good enough, the opinions of other people are none of my business, if they are good they go to my head and feed my ego, and if they are bad my ego feeds the opinion and takes negative presence with the ego. My past is not my potential.

How will I always remember that my value is given to me by my creator' not other people?

I had to learn true approval comes through the spirit in the quiet where I live my values.

How do I know what my values are? When I'm alone do I have Integrity? Am I always honest? Decide your values?

Religion was like a map, tangled, and a way to get to a place that was another destination. A place to the future or a reminder of the past. The rules and entanglement of people. Places, and things, for me the rules were rigid and left me feeling separate from God, the truth is I am not separate from God and God is not separate from me. We are one.

What path do I want to take? It is okay to change direction as long as you have one.

I did not turn out to be a size 2, I turned out to be me, happy, loved, healthy, vibrant, and alive. And I am perfect.

How will you except your perfect body as it becomes thinner and takes on its own natural form, (your shadow is a clue to that physical form.) How will I accept how my creator made me and reveals me?

I am open to the miracle of my life. The miracles in my life and I am grateful I did not leave before the miracle happened, the miracle of knowing.

How will you commit to yourself with all you learned through your journey of miracles?

Spirituality is where surrender happened, I was knowing my connection to God, my oneness to God, my purpose through God, my love for life force and life itself, where I feel the power of God in every whisper in every silent moment, in every blessing, in every bit of gratitude and appreciation, in every breath I take, in every tear I shed, in every moment of appreciation. This is real to me. This is where I choose to live.

What are you willing to do? Keep asking that to find the answers when you don't know the answer.

This is where I feel my pulse in the morning when I wake, and awe because I woke, I find thankfulness in my day in this present moment, beauty in the words and sounds of my beautiful world, kindness, and understanding for others in my heart, understanding for others as they grow and go their way, where I hear the song of my own Soul. I have a divine understanding of why a caged bird does sing, it sometimes wants, but mostly because she must.

QUESTIONS TO ASK MYSELF AND JOURNAL ABOUT:

Have I forgiven myself yet for the damage I caused myself and others?

Can I react in a way that will not hurt myself, others, or my body today?

What will I forever do differently because I completed this book? Have you surrendered to what you have no power to change.

Are you willing to change what you can change.

Are you willing to seek out the differences between people and know that all the right people are in your life.

Are you grateful for your life every day? Are you appreciative of others every day?

Now that you know that binge eating did not solve your problems or your fears it only made you fat and unhealthy, and unhappy, what will you do instead to relieve stress?

EPILOGUE

The Ego and the Soul

It is not how I judge another that matters; it is that I judge at all.

It is not why I blame another; it is that I need to blame.

It is not how I justify it; it's that I need to justify it at all.

It is not how I was punished; it's that I punish.

It's not how I seek approval; it's that I need approval.

It's now how I seek perfection; it is that perfection is needed.

It's not that I have memories; it's what I do with memories.

It is not how I am responded to; but how I respond to others.

It's not what that I did things with or to my body; it's remembering I live there today with love.

It's not how I once screamed; it's the voice of silence that speaks the loudest.

It's not that sadness was here; it's that joy is restored.

It is not how I was criticized; it's that I chose to criticize.

It's not that we married; it's that we thought it was a requirement.

It's not how afraid I was; it's how courageous I AM. It's not how I have been shamed; it's that I chose to keep shame.

It's not how I became guilty; it's that guilt has no purpose.

It's not how I hide my light; but how I let my light shine.

It is not how I see myself; it is why I see a piece of God in myself.

It is not the suppressed energy; it is the renewed energy.
It is not how you learned; it is your willingness to learn a new way.

It is not what you believe you are; it is what you believe you can be.

It is not what you are ashamed to do; it is what you are called to do.

It is not what others intended for you; it is what your intention is.

It is not that we waited; it was that you showed up.

It was not the depression; it was the actions that renewed our spirit.

It was not how I was suppressed; it is how I rise up out of the ashes.

It is not how we were yesterday; but how we chose to inspire today.

It does not matter how we received the scar; only that we recognized the blue pearls in the soft tissues.

It was not that I did everything I could; it was realizing there was nothing I could do.

It is not what you believe you can't give; it is what you chose to give.

It is not the religion you experienced; it is when you let love become your religion.

It is not how you came to hide; it is how you heal and reveal the presence of God as your light.

It is not how others see us; it's how God sees us.

Perfect.

Written by the Author- Echo Laymon Pelster

The End

Echo Pelster is one of America's Most Sought-after Keynote Speakers and Coaches, she offers Only Forty Dates each Year.

She is the perfect Speaker for your next Meeting, Breakout or Event.

www.echopelsterspeaks.com

Made in United States
Orlando, FL
07 December 2023

40220737R00124